Biddy McGee
“God Help Us!“

by Bridget Shaffer

Order this book online at www.trafford.com/08-0278
or email orders@trafford.com

Most Trafford titles are also available at major online book retailers.

Note for Librarians: A cataloguing record for this book is available from Library and Archives Canada at www.collectionscanada.ca/amicus/index-e.html

Edited by Cynthia Sherman Ny.
Cover Design by Autumn Bernhardt
My Family's Input: Thomas, Bobbie Jo & Gary, Kelly, Colleen, Linda, Mary, John & Jeanne.
My sister Patty could not be there to add her input, because she was at another hospital dealing with a life and death situation of her own with her husband Doug.

ISBN: 978-1-4251-7259-6

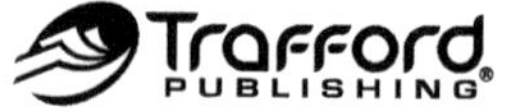

www.trafford.com

North America & international
toll-free: 1 888 232 4444 (USA & Canada)
phone: 250 383 6864 • fax: 250 383 6804
email: info@trafford.com

The United Kingdom & Europe
phone: +44 (0)1865 487 395 • local rate: 0845 230 9601
facsimile: +44 (0)1865 481 507 • email: info.uk@trafford.com

10 9 8 7 6 5 4 3

Dedication

This book is dedicated to all the people who un-selfishly made the decision to donate their organs so someone else can go on living. And to my own **DONOR, Thank you** from the bottom of my lungs for giving me a chance to breathe again. You will forever be in my heart even though I had never met you. But I look forward to our meeting when it's my turn to go home.

I would also like to recognize the **"Lifesource"** organization for their outstanding achievement in getting the word out that organs are needed, and for keeping the database with people who need a Transplant, and people who are Donor's. Without your efforts most of these transplants would not be happening. Thank You for all your dedicated hard work!

I also want to recognize the **University Of Minnesota** for all their great work, and for having such a dedicated team of Doctors working with me, who really do care about me. Also, for taking care of all my setbacks and problems that arose. Without your efforts I wouldn't be here today. I would like to give Thanks to my surgeon **Dr. Red** without her knowledge and skill I wouldn't have survived, also to **Dr. Black,** for backing up Doctor Red after my surgery. I would also like to thank **Dr. W** for taking great care of me while he was on rotation, and filling in for Dr. D. I especially want to thank **Dr. D** for me still being alive today. Unfortunately for him, I am one of his patients. He has always been so patient and kind even when I've done some of the dumbest things to myself. (He sure does hide his snicker well!) He sure has chosen the right profession to be in. The University is very fortunate to have such outstanding Dr.'s on their staff, and so am I!!!

Last, but not least, I would like to thank my family and my siblings for all their support through all of this. I know most of them were in agreement with this, but I know they were as terrified as I was. I LOVE all of you, with extra kisses and hugs to my husband, all my girls, and my son (the outlaw)!

PREFACE

We are all faced with choices that we have to make every day of our lives. Most of these choices that we make daily are minor. Then we have the major choices that could alter the way we are now living our lives. Some of us are faced with life choices that are not as easy to make, and require a lot more thought to be put into them.

I was faced with such a life choice after my last hospital stay in 2005. I had really bad lungs for most of my life (TB, ASTHMA, and COPD) and I was hospitalized five times in 2005 for infections in my lungs. The last episode was the worst and I was sent home on oxygen, to live out what time I had left of my life. As time went by, I could tell I was getting weaker and weaker all the time. After a couple of months, I decided that I wasn't just going to lie here and wait to die.

My doctor had mentioned a lung transplant to me, and so did my sister Linda, and my daughters. So I decided that if I really wanted to live I had better find out what if anything could be done. I went online and I read as much as I could about lung transplants. I realized that this choice wasn't going to be any easy one to make. I received a lot of advice from my loved ones, but I knew I had to be the only one who could make this decision. I weighed all the pros and cons, and I'm afraid I came up with more cons than pros. It was such a tough decision and I didn't think I had the courage to make this decision.

As I lay in bed one night worrying about all this, a serene calm came over me, and I decided that I couldn't leave my family yet, and that I wasn't through with this life yet. My mother came to me and whispered softly into my ear:

"Please listen very close to what I have to say,
Don't worry about death and look the other way,
Make your decision, to live another day."

When I awoke the next day, I told my husband that I had decided to have the transplant because I was no longer feeling afraid.

While I wait for a lung transplant, my sister Linda suggested I keep a Journal of my thoughts and feelings. I can't say you will actually call this a journal, but it will definitely be my feelings. Every story has a beginning, but I'm not quite sure how to begin mine, because it doesn't actually start at the beginning. I thought that once I picked up a pen, the words would magically appear on the paper. I have so much I want to say (and believe me anyone who knows me knows that I'm never at a loss for words), but I'm actually having trouble putting my thoughts into words for the first time in my life.

As I sit here reflecting on my life, I am remembering that I really did have a great life, and I'm remembering a lot of things about my life as I actually remember it, or what was told to me. I chose to call my journal "Biddy McGee" because my grandmother used to say this all the time, "Biddy McGee God help us," and unfortunately, she was referring to me. But this will actually be explained at a later time in my journal. So now if you don't mind, I will start off in the present, and from time to time, I will go back and reflect on my past, so you can get a better understanding of me as a person, and of my family.

Chapter 1

I went on the lung transplant list on September 23, 2005. Just to go through the procedure to see if you even qualify for the transplant is a story in itself. It consists of a full week of tests and you are pretty exhausted by the time the week ends. I always thought that a lung transplant was something they did as a last resort, but the truth of the matter is you have to be in the best physical condition as possible to increase your odds of surviving the transplant. My lungs are shot, but the rest of me is in really good condition.

One of the many tests they do is called a "Gated Blood Pool Scan" that is where they draw your blood, and mix it with radiation, and then put it back in you to watch it go through your system. (I'm sure my husband was up all night waiting to see if I would start glowing in the dark after that one.) Another real pleasant test was called an "Esophageal Manometry" in which they put a tube down your nose to look at your esophagus, and then they insert a smaller tube, which is connected to a device that measures the amount of acid produced when you eat. You are to eat three meals, then they remove it after 24 hours, and they have the results recorded in the device. That was one I really didn't care for. I tried to pass on it, but it was required, so no such luck. The technician said this was a more advanced procedure than the old one, but when I had an ulcer, I had the old one done about four times, and the only unpleasant part is when they have you swallow the tube, but you are partially sedated, so it wasn't bad at all. With the new one, I even choked on a piece of lettuce because it got caught on the tube. So, DON'T EVER eat lettuce during this test. It really didn't hurt at all, but it always felt like there was something stuck in your throat. (I will most definitely run in the opposite direction if a doctor suggests I have this done again.)

The only really other memorable test was the "Heart Catheter." The doctor that did it was very nice, and he explained what they were doing at all times. He had jokingly asked me if I had ever been a model, and since they inserted the tube in the groin area, I thought he was referring to my chicken legs, but he was actually talking about my arteries (he said they were so good, they could be on the cover of vogue). TOO BAD, the people at work were always commenting on my chicken legs, so I thought I would call there and rub it in, but I guess I won't mention this to them.

There were many other tests during this week's time, but I really enjoyed going to the Transplant Support Group. I was able to talk to a lot of people who were going through the same things that I will be going through, and most of them said that there were a lot of set backs, but they would do it all over again if they had to. Just to be able to breathe again was such a wonderful feeling. I haven't been able to breathe well in such a long time, I don't know what it will feel like, but I'd like to give myself the opportunity to find out.

Chapter 2

Today is Friday October 7, and my feeling right now, is that I have so much I want to get done before I get called in for the transplant. Along with everyone else, I'm a procrastinator, so I haven't even started but a couple of things.

I want to finish putting together my family photo albums. I have one for each side of the family, but mine has a lot less pictures in it than my husband's side. We are a very close family, but obviously we are very stingy or cheap with our pictures to each other. I have four sisters and one brother, and most of their children are grown, married, with children of their own. I am missing a lot of photos of my nieces and nephews when they were growing up. I am also missing a lot of their wedding photos, and I need pictures of their children. So my first priority is to write them each a letter (I suppose a phone call would be faster) and get some pictures sent to me. I can hardly finish this project without these photos. I, on the other hand, have about 30 photo albums of my children and grandchildren growing up, but I am also bad at sending off pictures to everyone. That is why I have so many photo albums.

Second, I am working on an afghan that I'm making for my best friend (Karlyn) for Christmas. I would really like to finish this, so I'll keep working on it until I get it done. Since I was so sick this past year, I had a lot of lay around time, so I made each of my children, grandchildren, sisters, and brother an afghan. I'm hoping that when they use it, they fondly remember it came from me. To tell you the truth, I'm really sick and tired of making Afghans, and I need to give my fingers a rest. Well that didn't work as well as I expected. My daughter and I took a run to Wal Mart, and I found a really colorful yarn that would make a gorgeous afghan, so I bought some. I really am a glutton for punishment. It's like an addiction, once I get started I have trouble stopping.

I also want to write a letter to each of my children and my husband to let each of them know how much they meant to me in my life. But I keep putting it off, because each time I started a letter it sounded like a good-bye letter and I don't want to be saying good-bye to them. But I want each of them to understand the wonderful qualities that they each possess, and how they helped me get through with life's ups and downs. I know my surgery can go either way, but I don't want to think about the possibility of not surviving it. But, if I don't write these letters, I will be kicking myself to hell and back when I'm gone! It is so hard to write such an emotional letter, but it will remain on my things to do list until I get it done. I will re-address this issue when I'm emotionally ready. (Funny I should say to Hell & Back)!

I'm also trying to get my affairs in order. My husband has never had to make out the bills, so I have put a monthly pay chart on the computer for him, and it explains what each bill is, what amount has to be paid, and the date it is due. I also made copies for 2006. I also made him a list of everything that is in the safety deposit box, including my insurance policies that he will need if something happens to me. He is trying to avoid this subject, but my girls know where I keep this information, so they will help him through the adjustment period. Things like this are very important to be done, but no one wants to think about the possibility of death. Actually, I don't either, but being prepared really helps your family. I know a lot of people even pre-plan their funeral, but I'm not ready for that yet. Maybe when I get worse I could handle it, but my thought right now, is that I still have a lot of living to do.

I want my house to be sparkling clean. This is something I cannot do because of my lungs. I have to rely on help to get this done. My sister came over and helped my daughter clean my windows for the winter, so at least that part has been done. But I'm a very impatient person so to me this part hasn't gone fast enough. Remember how your mother always told you to wear clean underwear just in case you get into an accident (like the doctor is really going to notice when you are lying in a bed covered in blood if your underwear are clean), well I feel it's also a reflection on a person as to how well they take care of their home. My mother was a cleaning fanatic, and unfortunately for my family I inherited this trait from her. But as you could probably guess I'm not having a bunch of people jumping up and down to volunteer to do this. Even if they did, I'd probably think they had a screw loose, because I've never heard anyone say (Yippy I get to clean my house today), if I did, I'd suggest they go get psychiatric help.

So as you can see, I have a lot of things I want to get accomplished, and my wait for the transplant could go either way, fast or slow, because I have AB+ blood, and I'm the only one on the list with this type of blood. But it could also mean that I could be waiting quite a long time for a match. I really want this transplant, but I'm not as ready as I actually thought I was, because I have so much I want to get done first.

Chapter 3

I guess you can say I fought just as hard to come into this world, as I'm doing now to stay in it. I was the first delivery for a new obstetrician, and I would or could not come out. He thought that my mother wasn't pushing hard enough, so they dressed my dad in a mask and gown, and had him go into the delivery room to try and talk her into pushing harder. She explained to him that she was doing the best she could but that something was wrong, the baby just would not come. The obstetrician finally figured that there had to be something wrong so they chased my dad out, and the doctor checked and found that the umbilical cord was wrapped around my neck, and that every time she pushed, it wrapped itself tighter. He reached in and unwrapped the cord, from around my neck, and I came out a nice purple color!! They kept me in the hospital for a couple of weeks in an incubator before they let my parents take me home. I had to fight to come into this world, and now I'm fighting to stay in it.

My parents already had a daughter, and they were expecting a boy, so I went home with the name baby girl. My dad thought he would do a great tribute to my grandmother (my mom's mom) and ran down to the courthouse to name me after her. Her name was Bridget, so that was the name that he picked out for me. He should have talked to her before he did it, because she actually hated her name, and had it changed years later!! **(Go figure)!** I actually liked the name, because I was Irish, and there was a saint named Bridget so I thought when I got older that I actually had a cool name. Besides I never ran into many Bridget's in my lifetime, so it was actually kind of unique. I suppose I had better be thankful that he didn't name me after my mother (her name was Agnes) or I would have gone and had it legally changed!! Where do people come up with some of the names they pick for their children? "Agnes," how or why would anyone ever pick that name!! Even she hated it, she actually never went and had it legally changed, but she decided to go by "Ann Marie," because she really liked that name, so no one called her Agnes, they called her Ann Marie. Talking about weird names, my dad's name was "Cecil," excuse me, but who in their right mind would name a child Cecil? When we were kids growing up, the only other time I heard that name was from a cartoon called "Beanie & Cecil." We always harassed my dad after that asking him where Beanie was. He didn't think it was as funny as we did , and I think the joke got old really fast, but you know how kids love to tease so we kept it up relentlessly until he threatened to do us bodily harm!

People really ought to take the time and think about the name they are giving their child, because it will be with them all their life. Do the child a favor, and don't name them after a distant relative (just to pay honor to them), the relative won't know, so let the name stay dead & buried with them, especially if they didn't even like their own name!

Chapter 4

It's now Monday October 10, and it has not been a very good day. My coordinator at the university called and said that they are temporarily taking my name off the transplant list, because the lung culture is still showing positive for a strain of TB. They said that they have been growing this culture since I gave it to them in August, and they still haven't been able to identify what type of strain it is. The lung specialist has now decided that he will turn it over to an infectious disease specialist, and see if they can work with the culture to see what will kill it (if anything). She said once they find the antibiotic, they will immediately put me on it, and I will continue to be on it until about a year after my transplant. The concern they have, is that once they suppress my immune system, if this disease is not being taken care of, it will attack my new lungs and destroy them. For some reason my immune system is keeping it from harming my lungs farther, (so they say) and that this is not a big problem so not to worry about it. They hope to have an answer in a week or two!!

Well, maybe for them a week or two isn't a long time, but for me it seems like a VERY LONG time. The real reason this is bothering me is that I knew TB had a part in destroying my lungs, and the first question I asked during my testing was, "Would this bacteria try and destroy my new lungs?" I felt that I didn't want to put myself through all this testing for nothing if I could never have a transplant. They told me that it would not be a problem because it was not active!! Well how would they know that, I can never have another test because I was positive!! I guess at this point all I can do is sit and wait, and hope for the best. The infectious disease specialist confirmed again to me that this was a temporary setback, and that they will be able to fight it with some type of antibiotic. I sure do hope so. In the meantime, all I can do is wait to be activated on the transplant list again. What a Bummer!!!

Don't you just wish your brain would shut itself off at night, so you could get to sleep without thinking of everything? I was thinking again about this infectious bacterium, and that they have known about it since the end of August when I first went to the university for testing. They said that since they could not identify it, they will try and find out what will kill it. I don't know what you are thinking right now, but my thoughts are if you don't even know what it is, how you could possibly know what type of damage it is still doing to my lungs. And what happens if you can't find anything to kill it? Does that mean that eventually it will kill me? Bad thoughts! Bad thoughts! There I go again, with negative thought waves…I have to think positive…or else it will begin to drive me crazy. Patience once again is not a virtue I was born with.

Chapter 5

Back to my life after my birth – it was about as normal (or abi-normal) as you could expect anyone to have. I came home to an older sister who wasn't quite sure she wanted me there or not. She must have decided that she didn't like me, or she was trying to see if I was actually real, because she reached into my crib grabbed my finger, and took a big bite of it. After a scolding from my parents, she must have decided she'd just ignore me, because my parents said she didn't pay much attention to me after that.

When I was about 10 months old, my mom had me outside on a blanket with her, when she ran inside to get something; the neighbor boy who was cutting his grass came too close to the blanket, and almost took one of my toes off. Thank God power mowers hadn't been invented yet (or if they were no one in my neighborhood could afford to buy one). So that was my first trip to the hospital. Have you ever seen the movie "Horror Hospital," well that's what it was like to go to that hospital. It was very large and scary!! Of course I was too young to remember that trip, but I was there many times after that, and I would have rather stay home and live with the pain than to go to that hospital.

When they finally decided to close that hospital, it was like they up and abandoned the place, because they left almost everything there!!! I know this from not actually being there, but it was a favorite hangout for my daughter, her friends, and a couple of her cousins that I was told about years after the fact. Of course there was no electricity but they always bought flashlights with them. They checked out the whole place from top to bottom. They said there were so many rooms and hallways it was unbelievable to them. They said their favorite thing to do was to have wheelchair or gurney races up the halls. The halls were so narrow, you could touch each side with your arms to help you push. The last thing they ever did was to go down and investigate the morgue. They knew it was in the basement, but they never had enough courage to go down there. They remember that they had a tough time opening the doors (a vacuum must have been created because no one was going in or out of there), and when they finally did get the door open, the first thing they noticed was that it had a strong medicine smell. When they started to investigate and opened up the refrigerated doors, it dawned on them what was kept in there and they all ran up the stairs and never returned to the hospital to play again.

Reminds me of a story my uncle told us about working for that morgue. He said one of the guys who worked with him, was terrified of dead people (not quite the perfect career choice for him I'd say) and they liked to tease him. One day they were called to bring a deceased person to the morgue. When they were in the elevator and the guy was in front, my uncle decided to sit the corpse up. The guy turned around after my uncle said something to him, and he screamed and left claw marks on the elevator doors from trying to get out!! My uncle apologized to him, because he never really thought he was that scared, and from then on, he worked with this guy to help him cope with doing his job. If it were me, a career change would have been better. But he stuck with it, and knowing my uncle, I'm sure he still harassed him every chance he got no matter what he tells us.

Chapter 6

Today is Friday October 12 and I still haven't heard back from the university. It is starting to get on my nerves. I don't understand why they haven't found an antibiotic yet. I called my lung specialist, because the last time I was hospitalized, it was a lung infection, but he said nothing grew from their sputum culture. They just treated the bacterial infection and I did get better. I think the University has too many patients, and not one individual is important to them, plus the co-coordinators work with too many people, and it takes a while for them to address an issue that comes up for you. But it suddenly has gotten very important to find out why they don't feel it is that important to be treating me now!

But on a brighter note, I finished Karlyn's afghan so I know that she will be getting a Christmas present that I made especially for her. I also started to make a new afghan with the new yarn, and it is very hard to work with. It might be great colors, but the yarn separates too easily, and anyone who crochets knows what a pain that is. But I'm not making it for anyone in particular, so it doesn't matter how long it takes me to finish it. Of course no one else in my family crochets, so if the surgery doesn't go well, it will either be a scarf, or a table runner. I also started to put my family album together. I have to still call them for pictures because there are a lot of blank pages, and the only talent I have with drawing people, is that I draw great stick people.

Chapter 7

Coming from a family of six children, we spent a lot of time playing with each other because we were all really close in age except for the youngest two. We had a lot of our own friends, but it was also just as fun to hang out with each other. You might say we were friends, besides being family. Some of the things we did, I'm really amazed that we are still all alive today. One of our favorite things to do was (dad taught us this one) to go upstairs and get all the blankets from our beds and make a maze with them. We would hang them on the clothesline downstairs in the basement and run through the maze. We even had some closed off, so you had to back up and go another way. We would turn off all the lights, and one person would try and find everyone. Something like hide and seek, but if you were real quiet, they could walk right past you, and not even know you were there. We would spend hours entertaining ourselves with that one. I wasn't there when this happened, but my brother told me that when my sister Patty was the person to find everyone, she would clunk you with a baseball bat to let you know that she found you. She had clunked my brother a little too hard and she about knocked him out. While he was lying on the floor seeing stars, they were trying to decide what to do about him. Patty finally decided just to let him lie there and see if he wakes up. My mother used to tell us to stay away from Patty because she was a bit strange (now I know why she used to say that)!! We really enjoyed this game until the lights would come on, and you knew my mother found all the beds a mess (she always made them daily). We had to put our blankets back on the beds, and my dad would be in trouble for teaching us that one.

We also really enjoyed scrubbing the basement floor; we would put lots of soap in the water, put our bathing suits on, and slide around from one end of the basement to the other end. That was GREAT fun. But I'm sure it was another non-favorite of my mother's because I'm sure she got stuck with trying to get all of the soap off the floor (she should have made dad do it because it was something else he taught us). We certainly had the cleanest basement floor in town.

Another one of our favorites, we had open stairs (no back boards) that went down to the basement. One of us came up with the crazy idea that one person would be under the stairs, and when they said "go," they would stick the broom handle out from under the stairs and we would all try to make it down the stairs before the person with the broom could trip you. Thank God we weren't very good at tripping someone because we had a cement floor, and that would have been very bad for the person who could have fallen down the stairs and hit the basement floor. But we were kids, and all we knew is that it was a lot of fun, and we never thought about the bad consequences of that game.

Another thing us older kids did was to scale the outside of a bridge. HOW STUPID, if you ever fell, you wouldn't be alive to realize how dumb it was. But we did it for fun, or because someone dared us to. That was until we heard that two brothers had fallen, or one of them jumped off the bridge when the other one that had fallen never resurfaced to save him (they figured one or both hit their head on a boulder under the water). Both brothers ended up drowning. They were kids we knew and had played with, but they never were with us on our bridge scaling escapades, but no matter why they did that, we never scaled another bridge again! It was a very disturbing reality to see the pain on their parent's faces, and realized that we could have put our parents through the same pain.

Chapter 8

Our home was the neighborhoods hang out. All the kids liked to hang out there because the biggest kid in the neighborhood (our dad) always played games with us. When he got off the bus on Friday afternoons, all of us kids were there to meet him, because he always bought us a bag of penny candy. Of course a lot of the neighbor's kids meet him there also, but we were HIS kids. And only we received a special bag of penny candy. However, the rest of them knew that as soon as he changed out of his work clothes, the fun would begin, and that he bought home candy for everyone.

We played hide and seek, had wheel barrel races, did tag team racing. He hid objects for us to find (like a scavenger hunt) and the last game of the evening was for everyone to take off their shoes, and stack them in the middle of the yard, my dad would mix them up, then when he said go, you had to find both your correct shoes, get them on, tie them, and be the first one back to the finish line. That person received a bag of candy. All the other games were rewarded with just a couple pieces of candy, so everyone loved the last game of the night. Needless to say, he only did this on Friday nights, so my mom got a little tired of kids coming to the door all week to ask if my dad could come out and play!!. I'm sure the neighborhood dentist loved my dad. I'm guessing that the parents weren't too fond of him, but who was going to say anything, or stop their kids from coming. It was free babysitting service for a few hours every Friday night.

Chapter 9

It has always amazed me that neither of my parents ever learned how to drive. In every other family we knew, the father drove, and in some cases both of the parents drove. Luckily we lived in the city, because we had to rely on buses to get everywhere. If we were in a real hurry to get somewhere (like a hospital) we usually took a cab if one of our relatives weren't available to drive us.

One day we were on our way home from someplace (I don't remember where) and my dad rang the bell for the bus to stop at the next stop. We all started to get off the bus. I was the last one out, and he shut the door on my foot. I started to scream and cry, and my dad ran back to me. The bus driver did not realize what he had done, because he started pulling the bus away from the curb. My dad ran along side of the bus holding me up, so I wouldn't fall under the wheels. With my dad and the people on the bus screaming at the bus driver to stop, it still took him two blocks before he stopped the bus. My dad was ready to kill the bus driver but he was so exhausted from keeping up with the bus that he didn't have enough energy left to fight. The passengers on the bus said the bus driver had a very rude attitude, and the bus driver told my dad that with our large family, we should be using the front door. My dad argued with him that is why they installed the mirror at the rear exit door, so the driver could see if everyone had gotten off. I suppose that the driver was partially right, but he was mostly wrong, and unfortunately my parents didn't have much money, so suing him was out of the question. However, I'd have loved to run into that driver later, because then I could have gotten the satisfaction of punching him in the face. SORRY MOM, if she was alive, she'd be telling me that violence never solved anything. But at least I would have had some satisfaction for myself.

Chapter 10

My parents were the type that never went out very much. They enjoyed playing cards, and my Aunt and Uncle would come over and they would play "500" on the weekends. Sometimes they would go to their house, but most of the time they came to ours, because then they wouldn't have to go back and forth to pick them up, then take them home. Weddings and funerals were about the only time they went anywhere. My mother would never have gone out and sat in a bar and drank all night. That just was not her thing.

One night they were going out (must have been a wedding) and I had gone down to the skating rink to occupy myself until it was time to go home. There were two little girls there who were just learning how to skate, so I thought I'd help them and hold their hands while they skated around the rink. They ended up getting tangled up, and all three of us fell down. I fell face first. We all got a good laugh out of it, and I continued to skate with them for a while longer. When I came in the door, my mom started screaming, and fell into a chair, my dad ran in to see what the matter was, and he ran and got a rag for my chin. I didn't understand what all the excitement was about, so I went in the bathroom and looked in the mirror. I had cut my chin wide open, but I guess because of the cold it didn't bleed much until I hit the warm air of the house. Boy did I get in trouble for that one. My dad called a cab to take us to the hospital to get stitches, and all I heard about on the way there was how I should have been more responsible. He acted like I did it on purpose or something because they were scheduled to go somewhere. He must have really felt bad once we got down to the hospital, because he fell over himself apologizing for what he had said. It didn't take us long at the hospital, and they were able to go out for the evening. But I was really mad at my dad and it was a few days before I forgave him for what he said.

Chapter 11

You know you hear about the physical abuse of kids, and I guess you could call what my dad did verbal abuse. He was just mad, and he wouldn't have ever done anything to hurt any of us kids, but at the time it hurt deeply. People should stop and think before they speak, to realize what it sounds like to be on the receiving end of what they are saying. I guess we all have said hurtful things to our children when we've been mad, but the realization of it just struck me hard!! Not then, but now!!

I know I haven't been the perfect parent, and I don't know anyone who is (I know a few that think they are) but words make quite an impact to all involved. They say kids are mean (and they are) but parents should just listen to themselves sometimes to hear what your child is hearing. Verbal abuse has always been here, and I guess I just never stopped to listen for it. So I decided that when I went to Wal Mart the other day, I would listen to adults having conversations with their children, and see if I could pick up on anything, here are some of what I heard, judge for yourself: "You are too fat to wear that type of outfit." "No more makeup you look cheap when you're wearing it anyway." "Why would I buy you that? You are too stupid to know how to use it." "Quit it, or your dad is going to beat you when he gets home." The parents might have been trying to get a point across to their child, but they sure went about it in the wrong way. If we each wore a mini tape recorder during the day, I bet you would hear a lot of stuff come out of your mouth, that you never thought you could or would say.

Well enough of this subject I'm acting like a psychiatrist, and I don't have a degree in anything. I just wanted to get my point across, but like I told you, sometimes I don't know when to stop. I stepped off my soap box now (or I should say my husband pushed me off), he said I got my point across, so ENOUGH ALREADY !!

Chapter 12

Today is Friday November 4th, so you can see it has been quite a while since I've written anything. I still haven't received an answer from the university. I'm sure they are really getting sick of me calling them all the time, but it has been two long months already, and I really expected an answer by now. They keep telling me to be patient, but I'd like to see how thin their patience would be if they had to wait for an answer as long as I've been waiting. I've been so depressed, I finished another afghan. You guessed it I bought more yarn to make another one. If I never do finish this journal, it will be because I can no longer make my fingers work.

It seems that when you desperately want something that is the time you want it the most. It's like when you have a car sitting in the garage, but you have a cast on your broken driving leg, so you cannot drive the car even if you wanted too. That is the time you really miss it. If you were able to drive, your car could sit in the garage and not bother you, because you have access to it any time you want!

Chapter 13

Here is a blast from the past again. Coming from a large family must have created quite a few challenges for our parents. When my older sister and I were old and curious enough, we went to our mother and asked her how come our brother was different from the rest of us. Back then, parents had such a hard time explaining sex to you. It was a taboo subject that they really didn't like discussing, but once the question was asked, an answer had to be given. She explained to us that we were girls, and he was a boy (that much we already knew) and that boys had "Doodle Bugs!" (Please forgive me favorite brother.) Of all the different words I've heard a penis called, where she ever came up with "Doodle Bug" was beyond me. Of course to two girls who had never heard what it was called before, this was quite a funny word, and we loved to tease him about it. Little did we know, other than my mom (who named it) no one else knew what we were talking about, so the joke was actually on us.

When we finally learned the truth, I swore that when it came time for my children to discuss sex with me I would never create a ridiculous name like that. I decided that honesty was the best way to deal with it, so when my girls were old enough to come and ask me, I told them it was a "pee-pee." Goes to show you how much more maturity went into my answer than my moms. NOT!!!

Chapter 14

My dad did part time Janitorial work at night to subsidize their income. A couple of us kids usually went with him, because you felt so grown up to be able to help vacuum and empty waste baskets. What my dad cleaned, was a construction office, which had a large garage attached to it, where they repaired their machinery. For a reward for helping, they had a pop machine in the garage, and dad would let us go down and get one when we were almost done.

I don't remember how the conversation started, but one night dad was telling us that the construction office used to be a funeral home. There was a set of stairs in the back of the garage, and dad said that down those steps is where they stored the bodies. One night when my sister and I went out to the garage to get ourselves a pop, we decided to go downstairs and see what was actually down there. Even though we were really scared, we turned on the light and headed down the stairs. My dad must have known that we would go exploring, so he waited until we were half way down the stairs, and he shut the light off on us. I don't think either of our feet touched a step as we flew up the stairs! Here sat dad laughing like it was the funniest thing he had ever done. Well he wasn't laughing anymore when we refused to go back there to help him clean anymore. My dad really was a great guy; he just had a morbid sense of humor sometimes. When he was there by himself, he had a spell where he couldn't breathe, and fell down the stairs. We were all so guilty about not being there with him, one of us always went with him after that. Plus my mother was so upset about what had happened she didn't give us much choice.

I'm sure raising six children there were a lot of unexpected trips to the hospital. The time we were playing tag downstairs, and a bike that was hanging on a hook (One of us probably put it there) fell off and landed on my younger sister Linda's head. Another trip to the hospital again. Another time we were playing tag there was an old chair sitting in the corner of the basement. When I ran by it, a spring that was sticking out of it went into my ankle, and came out about an inch above where it went in. When my mom came down, she panicked and instead of threading the wire out, she pulled it straight out and ripped the whole thing wide open. Once again, another trip we had to make to the hospital.

Chapter 15

When both my parents were hospitalized with pneumonia at the same time, they had a housekeeper come out and stay with us. They thought they had contracted the pneumonia from the bird we had. (But they didn't have to worry about getting it again, because my sister was trying to give it a drink of water by stuffing his head in a glass of water-you guessed it, he drowned)! She didn't know what to do with this bird, so she threw it up on their closet shelf, and my mother never found it for about six months. Dad was so attached to the bird so we told him the door was left open and he flew out.

After one day, the housekeeper decided that she could not take care of six children, so the youngest two were put in the hospital. (Not the safest environment to place two healthy kids). I don't know who made that decision, must have been the county. The rest of us hated this woman with a passion because of what she did, and because she was so mean!! We never ever would have talked back to either of our parents, but we sure did talk back to her. My older sister and I decided that we were not going to stay with her, so we started packing our bags to leave. She found out what we were doing and she came up the stairs after us. We threw our suitcases down the stairs at her. Needless to say, we were grounded to our room for the rest of the day. Halloween was the next day, and we were really looking forward to going out trick or treating, but the next day on Halloween she decided that we all had to stay home. We were all very mad about it, but there was nothing we could do, so I decided to pass out candy. That way, I could at least see all my friends. I was sitting on a stool with my legs wrapped around it, when kids came to the door. I was in such a hurry to get to the door, I forgot to untangle my legs, and

I fell flat on my face with the glass bowl in my hands. The bowl broke, and put a real deep cut in my wrist (a little more to the left, and people would have thought I tried to commit suicide.) We wrapped it in a towel, but it would not quit bleeding, and she would not take me to the hospital because she said that is what I got for not paying enough attention to what I was doing. (Letting someone bleed to death isn't a very responsible act either.) My sister snuck upstairs and called my Grandparents and told them that I was bleeding badly, and I needed to go to the hospital. Another trip to the hospital. But the bright side of this was we no longer had that housekeeper after that, and our two older cousins came to stay with us, and they were a lot more fun. A couple days later, my parents and the younger kids came home.

Chapter 16

When you get in your teens, you must leave your brain at home every time you leave the house. I was with a group of friends, and one of their older brothers came home, and asked us if we wanted to play a game that he and his brother started playing with his car. You were to sit on the hood, and jump off before he turned the corner to see if you could remain standing. And of course being the brainless wonder that I am, I decided I wanted to try it. Well when the time came to jump off, I got too scared to jump, so I stayed on and when he turned the corner I was thrown off.

At first I thought I just had a sore ankle, but as the evening wore on it was more painful. When I got home my mom wanted to know why I was limping, and I told her that I did the dumbest thing. I fell backwards walking up a hill, and landed on my ankle. (Either she was very gullible, or she figured I wasn't going to tell her the truth so why bother). In the middle of the night I woke up to the most awful pain I've ever had. I screamed for my parents, and guess what another trip to the hospital. When I landed on my ankle I broke the bone clean in half, so when I walked on it. It just went up and down, but stayed on top of the other bone, but when I was in bed the bones separated, and the swelling and pain began. I was in a cast for almost three months. You know, I could go on and on about all the trips to the hospitals, but when I started reading what I wrote, most of them were ME, so I figured I'd better quit while I was ahead.

They say people learn from their mistakes, but God forgot that sooner or later you hit your teens, and you are the only intelligent life form on this planet. We all have been through it, then we go through it with our own children. No wonder my mother used to say "Payback is a B----"!! She never actually said the word B----, but you got the idea. So to everyone out there who has a teen, May God be with you!! You'll need all the help you can get.

Chapter 17

My first love was when I was in the fifth grade. He was my fifth grade teacher. My mother told me it was something called puppy love, but I knew it was the real thing. All year I spent making sure I did all my homework, and paid extra attention in class. I studied real hard, so that when he asked for an answer to a question I could raise my hand and pray he picked me to answer it, to show him how smart I was. I drove my parents out of their minds; all I talked about from the time I got out of school to the time I went to bed was my teacher. I thought I would just die when summer vacation came, and I knew I wouldn't see him for three whole months. At first all I did was mope around the house, but when I started back playing with my friends again, we had a great time and by the end of summer if you had asked me, I would have said Mr. Who?? I had forgotten about the major crush I had on him.

My second love didn't come for a couple more years. Even though we grew up in the same neighborhood, and we knew each other, he was just one of the guys to me. Before they put 35E in outside of downtown St. Paul, that used to be all farmland, and there was an old barn that we really enjoyed playing in. Of course the owner wasn't too happy with us being there, so he always chased us away when he caught us. That old barn was where I found my second love. We used to climb up into the loft and take turns jumping out of the loft doors. Because we were young teens and just coming into the age of noticing the opposite sex, we made up the kissing game. The girls would sit on one side of the loft, and the boys would sit across from us on the other side. We sat across from the boy who was our age. We would then dare each other to crawl across the rafters, and kiss the person opposite you. The boy who sat across from me was my friend, but after my first kiss with him he became my second love.

The kiss was actually more of a peck on the lips (the way you would kiss your brother) but I was smitten with him. We played in the old barn quite often, until the farmer would come and chase us away. He actually shot at us with his rifle (I don't think he actually aimed it at us???) but it was enough to scare us away. I suppose he was trying to keep us out of it because it was very unstable, and not very safe.

Getting back to my second love, after that kiss I had dreams of us getting married and having lots of kids (Boy you sure knew how young I was to think something that stupid) and living in a nice house with a white picket fence. All the girls liked him, so he was never without a female hanging on him. I didn't care, because the kissing game was our secret. Then came the devastating news that his family was moving away. (My parents braced themselves for the storm that they knew was coming). I was heart broken, and I cried for weeks. My parents kept telling me that in time I would get over him, and of course I did, but at the time I thought my broken heart would be broken forever. But life goes on, and eventually I got over it.

The third love of my life was actually my first love. This was someone I really thought I'd be spending the rest of my life with. I knew that he had dated LOTS of girls, and I'm sure he had a lot of notches on his belt, but I really thought I meant more to him than that. We had our ups and downs as any normal couple would, then we'd get back together, but after a while I realized that love was not suppose to hurt as much as he was hurting me. I probably will never forget him because he was my first actual love, but because of our differences, we were not really suited for each other. I was not the type of person who could put up with his attitude, so eventually we drifted apart. My younger sister had gone on most of our dates with us, (because she wanted to go everywhere I went,) and he always said to bring her along. Eventually I think they both felt more than a friendship connection to each other, but neither one of them put it together.

I had met Tom (my husband) when my third love and I were still occasionally seeing each other. Tom was such a nice person, and I was attracted to him when I met him. There was just something different about him, he took me out all the time, treated me with respect and was very thoughtful of my feelings. We started dating, and he kept taking over more and more of my heart. We eventually married, and I realized that I was meant to be with him because he is my soul mate. We have been married for over forty years, and the reason is because of his encouragement, support, and Love. We both give and take in our marriage that is why it has worked for so long. There have been a few very rough spots, but we overcame them, and we prevailed.

Chapter 18

Guess what? Today is Wednesday November 9, and the university finally called me back. My Coordinator said that they still didn't have a positive answer, so they wanted me to see the infectious disease people. She said she talked to them last week, and told them they needed to schedule an appointment with me, but so far I have not heard from them. She said they needed to get more history from me, and then make a decision as to what should happen next. She said that if I haven't heard from them by the first part of next week to call her back again. She doesn't want me to get lost in the system and fall through the cracks!

I figure after waiting over two months already for an answer, I have partially ended up in the crack. But the most important thing to me is that I am still off of the transplant list, and I'm getting weaker all the time. Today is Wednesday November 16, and I still have not heard from the infectious disease people at the University. She was worried about me falling through the cracks, but with the rate this is going, I fell off the world! I just left her another voice mail telling her that it has been two weeks, and they still have not contacted me, so could she re-address this with them. I also told her that my husband is really concerned since it was bad enough to take me off the transplant list, and he wants me too definitely get a second opinion. Winter is so hard on people with lung problems, I'm just afraid I'm going to come down with a serious infection, and never have the opportunity to have the surgery and see what it is like to breathe! This has become very important to me, and I wouldn't want to miss out on it. All I can do is wait, and like I said my patience is wearing thin. Even if they never found a lung, it would not be as bad as not being put back on the list.

Chapter 19

When my Dad's mom was around eighty, she lived alone and whenever she wasn't feeling well, he always went and spent a couple of days with her, and my older sister and I would spend the weekends. She was a very nice and funny lady, and she had beautiful white hair that was down past her knees, that she always put up in a bun. We would help her wash her hair, then brush it, then she would twist it and put it up into a bun on top her head. She only had an extra room with a day bed in it, so one of us had to sleep with her, and we always fought about who was going to be first. It's not that we were afraid of her because we definitely weren't, but she said the rosary every night before going to sleep and it was kind of scary to lie in bed next to her and listen to her. Her hair would surround her face that she almost looked like an angel; it still was kind of spooky!

I had asked her if I could clean out her closets and drawers, because I was the snoopy one, so I could look at everything before I put it back neatly. One day she asked me if I could write her a short story, (I suppose she figured I knew how, because I talked so much). I was more than happy to write a story for her. (I think it was to keep me out of her things). So I started writing her stories. Every night when we lay in bed, she would read my story, or I would read it to her, and she would start laughing and say to me "Biddy McGee God Help US." Of course I never knew what that meant, and I never asked her, so I'd just laugh along with her. I continued to write her stories, she always read them, started laughing, and once again said "Biddy McGee God Help US." My sister and I were discussing this, and she never knew why Gram said it either, so I decided to look it up. Biddy is the diminutive word for Bridget, and McGee was my grandma's maiden name. So that is how I came up with the title for my Journal. "Biddy McGee" because that is ME!! (By the way, biddy means a hired girl or a cleaning woman) I guess it could be worse.

My grandma died about a year later, and my dad left it up to us kids whether we would go to the funeral or not. He described what would happen there (this was our first) so we ALL decided to stay home and remember her way she was. I should have asked for my stories back before she died, but when you are young you don't think of keeping written memories. It would have been interesting to read them (Because I don't remember any of them) and I would also like to know why she kept saying "GOD HELP US" after every story she read! With my imagination, I'm sure I came up with some very interesting stories, and it would have been fun to read them.

Chapter 20

When I was almost nineteen, my friend and I got into a car accident. She was about six years older than I was, and she had a young son that was at her mothers that we were on our way to pick up. It was raining and we were traveling on a road called Shepard road, it was very dark and curvy. It ran along side the Mississippi river. She was driving a little too fast for conditions (which she normally did) and I had to constantly remind her to slow down. We came to a bend in the road, and she lost control of the vehicle. We spun around a few times, and then hit the retaining wall that protected you from going into the river. We were both stunned for a minute, then we asked each other if we were o.k. and neither of us seen anything wrong with the other. (She really must have had glasses, and just didn't have them on not to have seen my injury). She tried to restart the car a few times, but no such luck. We sat there for a good fifteen minutes, and when no one else came by on the road, she decided that one of us should walk and get help. (You guessed it I was the young one, so I had to do the walking). Sure wish everyone had cell phones then, like they do today! So I took off walking, and she stayed with the car. I must have been in shock because I remember her telling me to go get help, but I don't remember much more after that. When I had left on my hike, the police showed up at the accident. She must have also been in shock, because the police asked her where the person was who was in the car with her, and she told them she was by herself. The officer explained that she could not have been by herself, because there was a big hole in the windshield on the passenger side. Then it dawned on her that I was with her, but she didn't know where I was. They put out an APB giving my description, saying that I had been in an accident, and I was probably walking around in shock. I do remember approaching a woman who started screaming and about jumped in front of a squad car to get their attention. The officers got out of the vehicle, and asked how I got that far from the accident in the time I did. Of course I had no clue, so they said the only way I could have made that good of time, is that someone had to have given me a ride. (To this day I shudder to think that I don't remember who picked me up, and how with the wound I had just dropped me off). The policemen helped me into the squad car, and then asked me if I knew how badly I was hurt. I said that I wasn't hurt, but they told me I had a big gash going down the right side of my face. When I reached up to feel for it, I put two fingers into it that was all she wrote, I passed OUT!!

When we arrived at the hospital, they called in a plastic surgeon to repair the wound, I did not come too until he was already working on stitching up my face. Even though I was nineteen, I asked a nurse if they could call my parents. When they arrived at the hospital they brought them back to see me, but when they seen all the bloody tissues on the floor around the bed, they were frozen and couldn't go into the room. They came out of their shock when they heard me ask if my parents were there yet. They came into the room, and my dad immediately started to cry (that was dad), and my mom asked me how I was doing. They had given me a lot of pain medication, so I told her I couldn't feel much of anything. The doctor explained to my parents that I was very fortunate. The wound started about an inch and a half above my eye, continued down to my eye, started again after my eye and went down for another inch. He said he could not explain why I hadn't lost my eye. To this day, I can still feel the crack in my forehead, and under my eyebrow the crack is about a half inch wide. It took over one hundred stitches inside and out to put my face back together.

While I was still being stitched, they brought my friend into the room to see what I had to go through, because she was having a fit about having to have a couple stitches in her chin. Well that was a bad idea, because it freaked her out so bad she took off out of the hospital, and a nurse and an orderly chased her to bring her back. When they finally caught her, they had to sedate her just to get the stitches done. When my parents brought me home from the hospital, my clothes were still covered in blood, and I still had dried blood over my face. My sisters thought I looked like Frankenstein! They were all terrified to have me sleep in any of their rooms. My little brother jumped up, and said he wasn't afraid of me, that I could sleep in his room. So for a while I had the company of my brother, because the girls avoided me as much as possible.

I looked in the mirror a couple of days later when I was braver, but I thought the plastic surgeon did a great job, because he had tightly closing the wound. It looked a lot better after I could wash off some of the blood, but until the stitches came out, the girls stayed away, because they said they had nightmares about me cutting them to match me. (Boy they sure had some vivid imaginations). My brother always held a special place in my heart after that, because he was the only one who actually was able to look past the scar, and know it was still me, and I hadn't changed, just my appearance was altered a little. He had the nickname Jackie growing up (I'm not quite sure why) even though his name was John. But to this day I call him Jackie he prefers to be called John, but I still call him Jackie. Love You Bro.

Chapter 21

When my father passed away, I thought my heart would never quit hurting. (I do believe there are people who actually die from a broken heart (the heart just can't take the pain and gives out). It was one of the saddest days of my life. My dad hadn't been feeling all that well, and he said he had a lot of pain in his lower abdomen. The doctor said it was possibly colon cancer, and he suggested surgery right away, to see if they could get as much taken out as possible. The surgery lasted for over six hours, and by the time the doctor came out to talk to us, we were nervous wrecks. He said that dad not only had colon cancer, but that the cancer had already spread through out most of his lower organs.

We were devastated to find out just how sick he was. After he was recovered enough to go home, the doctor came in to talk to him about setting him up for chemotherapy. My dad looked at the doctor, then looked at my mom and asked how long he thought that would prolong his life? The doctor said that he really couldn't tell him that, but without it, he only had a few months left. My dad chose not to have any chemotherapy done he said that whatever time he had left he didn't want to spend it being sick from the chemo. He wanted to spend as much quality time as he could with his family, plus, he told the doctor he hated hospitals, and would prefer to die at home. We had to take him back to the hospital about a month later, because his pain medication needed to be adjusted, so they put him in the hospital for a couple of days. While he was there, they called in our family priest to give him the last rites. When the priest showed up, a few of us were up in his room talking to him. When the priest walked in we were really surprised, because it was only my mom and us that went to church. My dad had never attended church with us (he said he had personal reasons why he stopped going). The priest knew that mom and dad had been married by the justice of the peace, because dad was a divorced man. He was telling my dad that he had do denounce my mother and live like brother and sister in order for him to be able to be given the last rites. For a man as sick as he was, I've never seen him so angry, he about jumped out of bed to go after the priest. We held him down, and asked the priest to leave. At this point we questioned our father, because as far as we could tell, they were already living like brother and sister. Dad had emphysema, and slept with the window open, and our mom had heart problems, and could not sleep with the cold air, so they slept in separate rooms. (We told him that we always heard one of them sneaking to the other ones room!!) But, we were all still kind of sad, because it would have been nice for dad to receive the last rites, so we each gave him our own last rites. He was able to come home after a couple of days, and with the new pain meds, he was still his amusing self.

He was always afraid of suffocating to death because of his emphysema, but he died peacefully in his sleep on March 21(he was only 62 years old). My sister was dating a guy that was a medic in the service (who was at my mom and dads house) and when they found dad Gary had tried to resuscitate him, but when he started pounding on Dad's chest I guess my mother wanted him to stop because she was afraid that he would hurt him. Because of his health conditions, dad could get very little insurance, so needless to say it wasn't going to cover his burial cost. Dad must have thought about this, because my sister and I went to the funeral home with mom to make the arrangements, and dad had already been there and had everything set up. We went down to the casket room to look at what he had picked out, and we just stood there in shock, because it was a cheap metal casket that looked like two laundry tubs pushed together!! My mom was in shock, but both Colleen (I keep forgetting to mention names, when I talk about my sisters) and I started laughing at about the same time because knowing dad, this was something he definitely would have picked out to save mom money. She threw a fit with the mortician, and told him in no uncertain terms that she was not burying him in a set of laundry tubs! We told mom that we would help her with the additional costs, because we were both working. She picked out a very nice looking casket that was not very expensive.

We had to get a sedan from them, because mom didn't drive and we needed a way to get from the funeral home to the cemetery. (It was a tight fit in my sister's car). The day of the wake, we all walked into the funeral home, went up to the casket, took a look and walked right back out of the room, because we thought we had the wrong room. The director met us in the hall, and mom asked where dad was. He brought us back into the same room that we had just left. My mom was very upset, because he didn't look anything like himself. She told him they should have asked for a picture, and he said that they don't like doing that because people tend to bring in photos of the deceased when they were younger, and that wasn't how they looked today. But mom said that at least they would resemble the person. What they did to my dad was to make him completely different. They thought that since my dad had been sick with cancer, his cheeks had sunken in, but he always had sunken in cheeks. They had used cotton to fill out his face, and he looked like the thin man with a fat face. Mom chased all us kids out of the room, and she stayed in there with them, and told them they were going to try and correct what they did. Of course there really wasn't much they could do at this point.

But for me, loosing my dad was so heart breaking it made it easier for me because he didn't look like my dad. We had met my dad's daughters from his first marriage, because they came up to the hospital when he was sick, but we had never met his son. My sister Colleen and her husband took mom to get her something to eat, and we were told to greet the guests coming in. The people we knew we greeted, but because this was our first funeral, we never said anything to the people we didn't know, some came up and introduced themselves, and others just paid their respects and left. When dads son walked into the room both my sister and I gasped at the same time he was the spitting image of my dad accept younger. Neither my sister nor I said a word to him; he walked up to the casket, stood there for a while, then walked out without saying a word to anyone.

Even though the wake was easier because he didn't look like dad, the funeral was Soooooooo hard. To have to say goodbye to someone you have loved all your life is the most difficult thing you will ever do. I can't even imagine that there could be a place called hell, because to me, that was like being in HELL that day. It was very hard to walk away after the funeral, because leaving him there by himself was so hard. Even though you know that his soul is no longer there, and it's just the shell of a body that it used, that didn't help to ease the pain. I never thought that I would ever get over losing him, but time does go on, and eventually it does get easier. I swore after that day, that I never wanted to go to another funeral, but my mom came from a family of fourteen, so the odds of that were impossible!

Chapter 22

I remember once my dad told us that when he came back to check on us, he would touch our feet to let us know that he was watching us. So usually, I managed to keep my feet wrapped up in the blanket, because even though I loved him greatly, I didn't want to have him touch my feet. Something about it just scared me.

Once, my youngest daughter lost her bearings on the way to the bathroom, and ended up in our bedroom. She was trying to feel her way around to see where she was, and she touched my feet. It woke me right out of a sound sleep, and I don't know who started screaming first, but it took my husband a while to settle us both down. To this day, my dad has never touched my toes, because I'm sure he knows that he would freak me out, especially after the last episode. But I'm sure he got quite a laugh out of that one.

My sister Linda and I both had our wedding arrangements already made before dad got really sick. We were both scheduled to be married in April the following month. He knew he wasn't going to make it to our weddings, but told us that we both were to go ahead with our plans. He felt that we had both made good choices for our spouses, and he was very happy for both of us. We both felt that since our weddings were the following month, he would still be here with us. But unfortunately he was right, he died before either one of us were married. Our little brother had to step into dad's place, because he was now the man of the family, and give us both away. My sister Linda was married to her husband Gary on April 3, and Tom and I were married on April 17th.

I guess now would be a good time to introduce you to the rest of the members of my family. From here on in, I will have to use factious names to protect my family's innocent spouses and children. When dad died, two of my sisters were already married. My older sister Colleen was married to her husband Frank; they had one son Frank Jr., and later had two more children, Gina, and Danny. My sister Patty was also married to her husband Chuck, and she had a son Michael, and then later had two more sons, Randy and Trevor. Linda and Gary had two children Angela, and Gary Jr. Tom and I had two daughters, Bobbie Jo and Kelly. My brother John (Jackie) and his wife Jeanne had two children Christie, and John Jr. And finally, our little sister Mary married Mark, and they had one son Mark Jr. All of us are still married to our original spouses, except my sister Patty. Her and her husband Chuck ended up getting divorced, and she later married Doug.

Mom liked us all to be together for the holidays, and with 13 Adults, and 13 children, we were getting to be quite a large group. Once our children grew up and started having their own children, we each started spending holidays with our own families. Now, one of us will have a holiday family party some time in January, and we all get together then. There are now over 40 of us, and we have a great time together, and have lots of wonderful memories.

Chapter 23

Today is Thursday November 17 my coordinator from the Transplant Center called me to say the she had an appointment set up for me with the infectious disease specialist on December 8. She said that he will be reviewing my history with me, looking at the results of the culture, and then making a decision as to how they were going to proceed. He could do one of a few options, put me on an antibiotic he thinks would work for a while, and see how it affects it, or just put me on this antibiotic and keep me on it until about a year after the Transplant. Or do nothing at all. Which will mean one of two things, it is nothing to be really concerned about, or because they could not determine how to treat it, they would have to take me off the list because they couldn't take the chance of this spreading to the new lung. This last part I don't really understand, because if it hasn't killed me by now, it cannot be that bad of bacteria (it may not even be a bacteria). But all I can do is wait until I see him, and hear what he has to say, and go from there.

But, my husband and I talked, and if their decision is to take me off the list, I will go to the Mayo Clinic for a second opinion. It sure couldn't hurt. Therefore, by December 8, I ought to be a nervous wreck.

Chapter 24

Today is Friday November 25, and it is the day after Thanksgiving. We all went to my oldest daughter's home for dinner. She had a wonderful meal, and we really enjoyed the day. I knew I was going to be spending the weekend, so I made arrangements to rent a portable oxygen unit.

We planned on going shopping on Saturday, and since I need someone to go with me, it was the perfect opportunity. The youngest daughter had to leave Thanksgiving night, because she had to go home to her dog. He had been sick, so she couldn't leave him alone for more than a day.

My husband our oldest daughter both had to work on Friday and since it is the busiest shopping day of the year, there was no way we were going to venture out. So I planned on being a couch potato for the day, and my son-in-law (that I will call Gary) was going to get out the Christmas decorations, and put the trees up and the lights on them. He waits until the wife and kids join him to put the decorations on. My son-in-laws father passed away a few years ago, and he had just moved into a new townhouse, and bought a Christmas tree (Artificial) to put up. My son and daughter decided that they wanted to keep his tree, and every year they put it up in the family room. He had it very nicely decorated with purple lights, and purple and gold ornaments.

My son put the first set of lights on the tree, and he was in the process of putting on the second string of lights, when half of the first one went out. The third one didn't even work at all. So he had to take them all back off the tree, and really regretted the idea that he had to run to target to get three new sets of lights. He came home with the new LED lights that are really bright and are suppose to cost only a few pennies to run, and last over twenty years.

But since they are new, they have a very limited choice of colors available, so he bought BLUE! We didn't have the heart to tell him that blue just didn't go with purple ornaments. Then to top it all off, the new string of lights didn't have as many lights on them, so he ended up running back to target, because he was a string short! When he finally got all the lights on the tree, he and the oldest daughter decided they might just as well put the ornaments on it, because it wasn't that big, and only had a couple boxes of ornaments. All the while they were decorating it, (the nice person that I am) was sitting on the couch harassing him about being color blind. I told him he wasted his money having the new eye surgery done, because he still needed his glasses if he actually thought the colors looked o.k. together. I sat there making smart ass comments to him, until he looked like he was ready to throw me out, so I laughed even harder!!! But truthfully, the tree looks very nice, but the purple ornaments have to go. He said just because he knows it's driving me crazy, he has no intention of changing the ornament color! He is such a nice son-in-law; I wish I had 100 more like him at home. (NOT!!!!)

On Saturday, my daughter and I along with the three Grandkids headed off to the Mall. After she went and got me a wheel chair, we were on a roll (no pun intended).We bought the girls along, because they are getting older now (two fifteen year olds, and an eleven year old).It is easier to have them try on two or three outfits at each store, then they leave the store, and I pick out the one I liked the best. It is usually the one they made the most comments about. We continue doing this throughout the mall, until I have purchased all the clothes. By the time we hit the fourth store, even though I am on oxygen I was getting pretty tired, so we called it quits for the day.

I need to go back out a couple more times to get the other stuff they asked for, but they usually give me a pretty good list to go off of. We went to a new Mexican restaurant for supper. It wasn't the greatest Mexican food I've ever eaten, but we were all hungry, so we ate it anyway. The men were on their own for supper, so they went out to eat by themselves.

Chapter 25

We have two daughters and spouses besides my three granddaughters. The older ones are our kids also, and deserve to get presents as much as the little ones do!! I even fill up their stockings. I am always harassing my oldest daughter's husband, because he is like a son to us, and we found some cute candy I am putting in his stocking. It has a small reindeer in the package, and it looks like reindeer droppings behind him, that are actually chocolate covered raisins. COOL!!!!

We were home about a half hour, when we received a call from my sister Mary, that Patty's husband Doug was in intensive care at St. Joseph's hospital with a massive staff infection. He had been in a different hospital prior to this, and had a hip replaced, which he never fully recovered from. They found him on the bathroom floor, and he was taken to the hospital by paramedics.

We left and went right down to the hospital. We weren't allowed to go into his room because they couldn't take a chance of him picking up anything else. My sister was the only one allowed in to see him.

Today is Wednesday November 30, and my sister still doesn't know very much more than she did the day he was admitted. He has an infection that has spread to his colon, liver, kidneys, and stomach. He is not responsive at all, but they said it was because he was in Toxic shock. He said it could go either way at this point, we're all praying he recovers soon and is able to pull through this.

Chapter 26

This must be taking a heavy toll on my sister Linda also. She lost her husband December 2 at the age of forty-one, and they never did find out what his infection was from. He had a cough that kept getting worse, so he went to the doctor for it. They said he had bronchitis. And gave him an antibiotic and sent him on his way. He still wasn't feeling any better after a week on the medicine, so they decided to admit him for tests, (this all began the first of October). He was admitted, and they said he had pneumonia, but they hadn't found out which kind yet. They put him in intensive care, and were giving him a lot of different types of antibiotics to see which one would work. After a week, they found he was getting worse, and they still hadn't identified the bacteria, so they wanted permission to send him to the University Hospital because they said that if anyone could figure out what was causing the infection they could.

By this time, he was so congested; they had to put him on a respirator to help him breathe. Because he was conscious he kept fighting the respirator, so they had to put him in a drug induced coma to give his body a chance to heal itself. For a few long weeks they ran tests, poked, and prodded, but still didn't know what caused the infection. The only thing they knew is his heart was throwing off vegetation that was causing his other organs to shut down.

Finally on the morning of December 2, my sister had a long conversation with his nurse, and she told her that he was basically being kept alive by all the medications. She called his doctor to confirm this, she also asked for a brain wave test to be done to see if there was any brain activity, and there wasn't so they decided to take him off all the medications, except for the IV and the respirator. He lived for only a short time after this. His heart just stopped beating, and he died.

My sister was so strong for her children during this whole ordeal. Gary was truly her soul mate and to loose him at such a young age had to be devastating for her, but she kept up a calm front throughout the whole thing. I truly admire her for being such a remarkable person, if anyone ever needs anything; she is the first one to help. She also said that since she suffered with Gary for a couple of months she knows what needs to be asked, and to be sure that the doctors are doing everything that they can for someone.

I think he received a lot of damage to his heart and lungs from breathing in Agent Orange in Vietnam. He was a medic, and he said there were some days that your whole body was literally covered from head to toe with this stuff. My sister had an autopsy done, but they were never able to identify the source that caused his death.

Chapter 27

Today is December 8, and I went to see the infectious disease specialist at the university. They were not able to identify exactly what is causing the bacteria in my lungs, but it is one of only a couple infections (TB is one of them) that it could be, so they put me on three different types of antibiotics, and when I go back in a month, they can possibly take me off one of these depending on if the new sputum culture I gave them can identify which one it is. I still have to be on them for a year, so it would be nice to only have to take one. The transplant team will review my case after the holidays, and make a decision as to how long I have to be on these medications before I can be put back on the transplant list.

Christmas was wonderful, my son-in-law made prime rib, and we had twice baked potatoes, with it. All the kids, big and little enjoyed opening up all their presents. Everyone received what they wanted, and we all had a lot of fun. Christmas is my favorite time of year. I hate the cold weather, but I really enjoy buying all the presents and putting them under the tree. Christmas was also a favorite time for my Dad. He was like a little kid who couldn't contain his excitement. He would wake up at the crack of dawn (sometimes earlier) and stand at the bottom of the stairs and start yelling "kids, guess who came last night"? My mother would be in the background yelling at him not to wake us up, but he would keep it up until all of us were up!! My parents never had a lot of money, but we always received the one thing that we really wanted, and depending on the cost we also received a lot of smaller items, but we all received the same amount of gifts. We used to use my dad's white socks to hang up for Santa, and it would be filled with candy, nuts, and an orange. Every year it had the same thing in it, but we all loved it.

I love decorating my house and getting it ready for Christmas. I love the anticipation of Christmas, but in one DAY it's over. The past couple of years we've started to decorate the outside. We never used to decorate outside, because we owned and lived in a four plex, and it was just too big. But now that we have downsized to a smaller home we started it, and we like to pick up at least one new outside decoration per year. We have everything set up on a couple of timers so they come on at dusk, and go for three hours before they shut off. We don't want to keep the neighbors up at night, we have one neighbor who already thinks we over decorate, and after many years of doing this we probably won't be her favorite neighbor.

Chapter 28

I went back to the infectious disease specialist today, January 12, 2006. He said that the culture I gave him in December did not grow anything so he took me off one on the TB medications. I still have to take the other TB medication (Rafampin) and the Ciproflaxin. He thought that the medication he took me off of was the one making me so sick to my stomach, so he said that I could quit taking the anti nausea pill, but after a couple days of being off the pill I started getting really sick to my stomach again, so I went back on them again. I had to give him another sputum culture, and they will give it six weeks to see if it grows anything again, and if it doesn't, I might be able to get off of another one of the medications.

But the GOOD NEWS is that I can go back on the transplant list, because they wanted me to be on the medication for a couple months, for it to be in my system, so it could not spread to my new lungs. I will have to call my coordinator to be sure I'm back on the list.

I also had better get going and start writing each of my kids and husband the letter that I wanted to write to them. I also want to re-do my will, so I had better get all this done and soon. For some reason I have become very nervous about the transplant and I wasn't before. Hopefully I settle down. I can see why my mother never wanted to have open heart surgery. It is very scary when you think about what they will be doing to you.

Chapter 29

This next story is almost unbelievable, but it did happen. My mother had rheumatic fever as a child, which damaged the valves in her heart. She needed valve replacement surgery, but she had a fear of dying during the procedure, and she didn't want to die that way, so she would never have it done. She had put it off for so long because of her feelings, that her heart specialist said that her heart was so bad, that now it was too late for Surgery to help. After a while, her heart was not working very well, that she was going into congestive heart failure, so he put her in the hospital, and told us that it was just a matter of time before her heart would stop.

Her lungs started filling up with fluid and on the EXACT same day that our father passed away, she went into respiratory arrest. We could not believe that, we were going to loose our mother on the same day!! They tapped the fluid from her lungs and per her on a respirator. We all knew the end was near, so we all took a leave of absence from work, and took over a room in the family waiting area. She survived that attack, and they moved her out of intensive care and into another room to wait it out. Our nightly ritual must have been very comical to the nurses on staff. Every night all six of us would put on our pajamas, robes, and slippers, and go to her room, to give her a kiss good night. All the staff knew us by name, so they paid no attention to what the visiting hours were if one of us couldn't sleep and we went to her room.

Mom was coherent so she knew all of us were there with her. After a few weeks, the respiratory specialist wanted to have a meeting with us. He felt that we shouldn't prolong the inevitable any longer, and that he suggested taking her off the respirator. One of us (I don't remember who) said to him "if we do that, wouldn't her lungs fill up with fluid and she will suffocate to death? He said that yes that would happen, but he felt it was inevitable, and we were just prolonging something that we eventually had to do. We all looked at one another, and said to him "but she's coherent"!! She will know what is happening to her. He said that yes she would. We told him that since she was coherent, that was her decision to make.

We left the meeting with him, and went to mom's room. I will never forget the look on her face and the doctor's face when we told her. It was total SHOCK. I don't think the doctor thought we could go right in there and tell her the truth. We asked her if she would like a second opinion, and she shook her head YES. My sister Linda called the University of Minnesota and explained to a doctor there what was happening, and could he help us. Their doctor said that they would send an ambulance to pick her up. The respiratory specialist was shocked that we were taking her out of this hospital, and going to a new one. The nursing staff was very encouraging to us, and told us that we were at least giving her a fighting chance. We took turns packing up all our belongings, and we were ready to follow them when they showed up to get her.

When we arrived at the university, they were already assessing her. After what seemed like hours, a doctor came out to talk to us. We will never forget this man. His name was Doctor Salmon, (not his real name) and he was the heart specialist. He told us that he was very positive that they could fix her heart, but he was very concerned with the fact that she had been sick and in bed for such a long time, that when he put her to sleep it would be permanent because she only weighed seventy-eight pounds!! We all went to her room, and Doctor Salmon explained all the pros and cons to her, and she looked at each of us individually for our opinion, and then signed for the surgery herself, so that none of us were responsible if she didn't survive it. They gave us time to be with her, and then they took her up to surgery.

Doctor Salmon told us that if we didn't see him for at least an hour, that was a good sign. Well, being the intelligent people that we were, we all decided that if we went somewhere else, he couldn't find us to give us bad news!! After being up in the cafeteria for a half hour, we decided that it wasn't going to work, and that if we were needed, that they could find us, so we went back to the waiting room. We met a really nice lady and her family in the waiting room. Her husband was in surgery getting the first heart and lung transplant that the hospital had ever done. So we all said an extra prayer to God for him to make it through his surgery also. (He did end up surviving the surgery and leaving the hospital before my mom).

Two of my sisters decided after a few hours of waiting that they would go back up to the cafeteria and get something to munch on. They got themselves lost, and ended up at the wrong set of elevators. When the elevator door opened, out came my mom with her eyes wide opened, and when they said something to her, she smiled. They came running back to the waiting room to tell us, and found that Doctor Salmon was there. He said it would probably be a few days before she woke up, and that we shouldn't be alarmed. My sisters told him about running into the staff bringing my mother back from surgery, and that she had her eyes opened. He was in shock about it, but he did say that she needed to sleep for her body to heal, and that he would make sure she was resting.

We all wanted to kiss him, but we didn't want to offend him, so we settled for hugs all the way around. After she was in intensive care about a week, one of the male nurses (they stayed right in the room with the patients) suggested that we set up a visiting schedule, because it was going to be along road back. We decided that he was right, so we made up a schedule where two people went at a time, and they would let the rest of us know what was going on. We are really glad we did it, because she was in intensive care for six months, and she had a LOT of set backs.

It was really funny to see her in the bed when you were coming up the hall. The nurses would brush her hair and stick it in a pony tail on top of her head with a decorated hair binder, and she would be lying there in her hi top tennis shoes. (They had us get her a pair of hi-tops, to try and keep the drop foot at a minimum.) She looked like a little kid with big feet!!! We would occupy her time by playing twenty one with her when they got her up in a chair.(She always won) I really like the way the university would have someone in the room at all times. You never had to worry about anything when you left the hospital. It was a very stressful time for both her and us that we didn't need to add to it.

After she had been in intensive care about six months, during one of our family and hospital staff meetings, they suggested that we start looking for an extended care facility to bring her to that could handle a respirator, because they felt she had been on it for too long, and each time they tried to lower the amount of air she was getting, she could not tolerate it. We told them, that we did not bring her to the university to have her be sent out with a respirator, and that they had to either get her off of it, or instruct us on how to take care of her. They said that it was impossible to take her home on a respirator, so we told them that then they had to get her off of it. They sent in a new respiratory therapist to work with her that was very young. He approached it from a different angle. Each Day he came; he would turn the respirator down (without her knowledge) and work on gaining her confidence. At the end of the week (We all showed up) he walked in and told my mom that he was going to be taking her off the respirator. She panicked, and told him she could not do it. He then informed her that he had been turning the respirator down daily, and that she was doing most of the breathing on her own. She allowed him to turn it off, and after a time when they realized she continued to breathe on her own, he pulled it. When he was done, he opened the door and told us that he was successful. We all let out a yell, and applauded him for his success.

When she was finally released from the hospital, she went to a rehab center to learn how to walk again, and be able to do things on her own. When she was released, she walked out on her own!!! We had her for 20 more years after that thanks to Doctor Salmon, and the wonderful nursing staff at the University Hospital. We also could not have done it without the support of all our husbands (in my brother's case, his wife) they had to take over the responsibility of being both the mother and father. They also had to do all the chores, all the cooking, and taking care of the kids. They even brought our families up to the hospital to visit us, and brought us up meals so we didn't have to eat hospital food all the time. I will always be eternally grateful that my husband allowed me to spend so much time with my mother, without making me feel guiltily about it!!

Chapter 30

I need to give you an update on my sister patty's husband Doug. He ended up being released from the hospital, and was put in a rehab center. They can do his daily dialysis right in his room. The doctor said it is going to be a long road to recovery, but so far he is doing really well compared to how he had been doing. I hope that my sister and her family find the strength in each other to deal with Doug's journey back to good health. My prayers are always with them all. He has fallen three times in the nursing home and broke the outside bone in his hip again. He was back in the hospital three times from the falls. He has finally started to recuperate some, he can walk with the walker but he will never be alright until he heals enough to go through the same surgery again to fix what the first surgeons did wrong. I feel really bad for the family because I can't be there to lend my support, but they know I don't get out much because of my breathing problems.

Chapter 31

I had to get out of this house for a while, so I ordered a portable travel oxygen compressor, and we went and spent the weekend of January 20-22 with my eldest daughter Bobbie Jo and her husband Gary. It is very rare that my husband ever has a full weekend off, so it was really nice to spend quality time with him. We went to Mystic Lake casino on Friday night, and the kids bought us supper. I had prime rib, and it was delicious. We then proceeded to go and play some slot machines. I won $125.00 on a nickel machine (that I cashed out), and my husband had to show me up by winning $170.00 dollars on another nickel machine (that he cashed out). Our son in law won $80.00 on a machine, and my daughter won $200.00 on a dollar machine that she cashed out. We divided up all our winnings, and then decided that we would only play for a while longer, and then we would go home because my son-in-law had to work for part of the day on Saturday. My husband and I continued to play slots, and my daughter and her husband decided to play pull tabs. My daughter won $1078.00 on a pull tab. She has a lot of luck!!

She has a pendent that she found at a Casino that she calls Mr. O'Lucky which has worked very well for her. She even let her boss borrow it when she went to Vegas, and she won quite a bit. I borrowed it to take with me when my sister and I went to the Casino, well it sure DIDN"T work for me, I wanted to flush it down the toilet!!

When she and I went to a different casino two years ago on her birthday she ended up winning $2000.00 on a pull tab!! Her husband took her to Las Vegas this past spring (her first time there), and she ended up winning over $10,000.00 dollars!!!! We ended up going home after she pulled the winner, so at least we came out with money in our pockets. My husband and I tease each other all the time that if it wasn't for our bad luck, we wouldn't have any luck. We didn't get home until almost 2:00 AM in the morning, we hadn't realized it was so late (I'm usually in bed before 10:00 PM) so it was quite a long day for me.

The next day we went to the Boat Show, we haven't been there in quite a few years. They had a lot of boats there, but the kids were interested in buying a pontoon. We have an older one, but they thought it was about time we updated! They bought a beautiful 23 foot pontoon that has a porta pot and a sink on it. It also has reclining Captain Chairs on the front, and the back has chairs for fishing. It has an L shaped couch, with a table that you can swivel, and a radio with a CD player. The best thing about it is that they are going to leave it up at our home, (because we have a house on a small lake) and we will be able to use it whenever we want. The only thing they asked for is for us to sell our pontoon, and buy a pontoon lift with the money. NO PROBLEM!!!

After we left the boat show, we had to pick up our oldest granddaughter (the youngest went skiing with her friends) and we headed to the Green Mill for supper. Once again we had an excellent meal. We spent the rest of the evening relaxing on the couch. The next day the kids made a wonderful meal for us, (my brother and his wife came over) and we left for home about 7:00 P.M.

When we moved, we headed North out of the cities, and when they moved, they headed south of the cities. But the drive isn't all that bad; it takes about an hour and 10 minutes with no traffic. With traffic it could take as long as two hours for them to head North on a weekend during the summer. But they will spend a lot more time driving than us, because we live on a lake home.

Chapter 32

My coordinator from the Transplant Center called me on Tuesday, January 24, and said that I am back on the Transplant list. I have to go and see the infectious disease doctor again on Feb. 23, so she made my six month check up with the transplant doctors for the same day. They take another chest x-ray; you have to do a lung function test with a six minute walk (not as easy as it sounds with bad lungs) then see the pulmonary specialist. At least I'll get it done on the same day.

I also scheduled an appointment with an attorney here in town, (for next week-Tuesday) to have a new Will made out I want to re-write mine, because some of the things are a lot easier on the ones we leave behind (if something should happen) if you put it all in writing, This way hopefully there will be a lesser chance of fighting being done over things. You know how it is whenever money is involved it could turn an angel into a monster! I still haven't met Karlyn for lunch, so I can give her the Christmas present I have for her. We had a date scheduled, but I had a bad day then, so we have to reschedule it. I better get going and give her a call.

Chapter 33

When I was finally put back on the Transplant list. I wrote my brother and sisters a letter. Here is what I wrote:

To my wonderful Siblings,

(Sorry it must be the drugs talking for me).

I wanted to write and let you all know what has been going on. As you already know, I went to the University of Minnesota for a Lung Transplant evaluation. That part is finally done. They put you through a battery of tests for a full week, and there is no part of your body that is not checked out thoroughly.

There are many tests, and some of them are kind of interesting. Especially the one they called a gated Blood pool scan. They take some blood out of you, then inject it with a radioactive material, then put it back into you, so they can see the blood going through your whole body. I was teasing Tom, and told him that I would be glowing in the dark for a few days. (I don't think he believed me, but I bet he was up during the night to check it out!!).

One of the things that are required in order to qualify is that you have to be in good physical shape, or they won't even consider doing the transplant, because you won't survive it. I always thought that was why they did it, because you were in such lousy shape! In one of the many, many, many, meetings they have you going through, they explained why this is required. The anti rejection and immune suppressing drugs really take a heavy toll on your body. It is not uncommon after a few years to need a kidney transplant also, because the drugs have ruined it.

I was very surprised to find out that the rest of me is very healthy. Usually the heart is taxed so much because the lungs are damaged, and they basically work side by side, but my heart IS IN EXCELLENT SHAPE. They figured that since I have been dealing with lung problems for so many years, that I have adjusted how much I needed to fight to breathe, and it just became natural for my system. But I really believe that working all those years on a job I really did like doing kept me active, and I adjusted to the progression of the disease. Now that I'm not as active I tire very easily. (Of course that could have something to do with the fact that I was hospitalized five times the past year.)

I met with a support group with the people that have had lung transplants, and even with all the set backs (and I guess there are many) they all would choose to do it again. I have started a list of pros and cons.

I have AB+ blood, and since that is rare, I could get an organ really soon, because right now there aren't any in the 5 state area that are waiting for lung transplants with my blood type. But like Tom said that could also mean that I could be on the list for quite a while because there are not very many organs available with that blood type.

My problem with making my decision right now is that Tom and I thought having a lung transplant would be our last choice only if it was between a transplant and not surviving. The odds are not the best, because a lung is very hard to transplant because it is very fragile. All the other organs are contained and protected within the body, but with a lung, you need the air to breathe, and sometimes it is very bad on people. The odds they gave us are:

1. 10% die within the 1st month of the transplant. (He said that is high, with the other organs its 1%).
2. 20% die within two years of the transplant.
3. 45% only survive for 5 or more years.

No one would give me an answer as to if I am problem free, how long could my lungs last as they are right now. If they told me 5 years, it would be a no brainier, and I'd prefer to stay the way I am. I have had much advice, but I know this has to be my decision.

The Transplant Center called, and said that I have been approved for a lung transplant, or possibly two. If both lungs are in good condition, and if no-one else on the list have the same blood type, they will give me both the lungs.

I have thought long and hard about this, and I decided to go ahead with the transplant if my insurance approves it. It was a very hard decision to make, but I want to be able to breathe again, and live a longer normal life if god is willing. It was too hard to explain all this to everyone, so I thought a letter would be easier. One of my employees wrote me a letter, and at the end of the letter he included this part of a poem, which says it all:

But he did promise strength for the day
Rest for the weary, light for the way
Grace for the trials, help from above
Unfailing sympathy, undying love!!

But look at it in a good way, if things don't work out, I'll see mom and dad before the rest of you, and you know how I like to be first, so I can tattle on the rest of you!!

Please take good care of my family, because they are going to need your love and support.

I love all of you very much

Bridget

This was a very hard letter to write, but I wanted them to know why I chose to have the Transplant done.

Chapter 34

My coordinator from the university called me today (Feb. 2, 2006) and said that they had another meeting regarding my transplant today. I was originally on the list for either a left lobe, or both lungs. They have decided that since they cannot take a chance with this bacteria hiding in the left lobe, they want to do a double lung transplant only. This way, they are sure that the bacteria cannot spread to my new lungs. I cannot decide if this is good or bad news! I don't know if I will have to wait longer to get the Transplant, or if it doesn't really make a difference since I am the only one on the list with my blood type. But it is definitely scary to realize that it could be soon! She once again warned me to be ready because she really thinks it will be soon.

Chapter 35

How come when you become a Grandparent, you worry more about your Grandchildren than you ever did for you own child? I think it is a control issue!! You had control over your own child, but you have no control over your Grandchild!! It's not that you don't trust your own child to raise their children, it's because you have NO say in the choices they make for their own children, and it bothers US!

I don't know how other people handle this, but for myself I have the hardest time keeping my BIG MOUTH SHUT! I think for myself, it's because I'm such a worry wart. My children used to tell people that I was such a worry wart; they couldn't even ride their bikes around the block until they were in HIGH SCHOOL! I know I was bad, (well we lived on an extremely busy street) but I don't think I was that bad. It was probably more like Junior High School. I always hear people who are in their mid forties to early fifties say they hope they don't become a Grandparent because they are just too young. Well if they are like me, I was married right out of high School, and I had my first child at nineteen years old. So needless to say, I became a Grandmother at forty-one! But unlike most people, I was ecstatic. I never felt like it was making me older faster!! I guess I'm not a vain person, because I was HAPPY!! I'm sure these people changed their opinion when they became a Grandparent for the first time. Or. Maybe not!!

When we found out our daughter was pregnant, we were hoping for a boy because we had two daughters, so it would be nice if it was a boy. Our daughter went into labor about a month early. They knew the baby was small, so they kept trying to stop the labor, (so the baby had a chance to get bigger) but after a couple of days of starts, and stops, they realized this baby wanted out!! So needless to say, when it came time for our daughter to push, she was exhausted and the baby would not drop down. The baby was in so much stress, that it had a bowel movement, and they moved my daughter from the birthing room to a delivery room.

They were only going to try and deliver the baby one more time, and if no luck, they were going to do a C-section. They had the pre-natal intensive care staff there, and when she delivered, they took the baby right out. We were told that this was happening, because it could be fatal if the baby swallowed any of the fluid. The baby was a beautiful little girl!! I do mean little; she was only five pounds, and was only twelve inches long. I had never seen such a small baby before! Everyone had said that her mother was small at eighteen inches, but it was hard to believe she was the size of a ruler!!

We were able to go into the pre-natal intensive care unit to see her, but we had to put a mask and gown on. In fact we seen her before her mother did! She was such a tiny thing lying there with snow white hair (what she had of it—not much) and such beautiful features. We were so proud to be Grandparents. We took a look around in the intensive care unit, and we could not believe our eyes. There were so many babies that were quite a bit smaller than her!! One of the baby's names was Mathew, and according to the note on his incubator, he was now at four pounds having come into this world a couple of months earlier at under TWO pounds. It was just un-believable that so many of these babies lived, thanks to the care and all the new technology available to the doctors. She is still a little person (she doesn't like to be called short) and she is going to be sixteen in July. She is a beautiful girl.

When our youngest daughter was pregnant with her first child, she wanted me to be her coach, so I was able to stay in the birthing room with her when she had the baby. This was actually the first time I had seen a baby being born. When I had my children there was a mirror set up in the delivery room, but the doctor blocked my view, so I couldn't see. It was a really neat experience to witness.

When she pushed the head out, the doctor turned the head, (opposite of the side I was on) and cleared out the mouth, I was kind of shocked to see all the blood. I guess I hadn't realized you bleed so much. When the baby was finally out, I thought I had a Grandson, and I screamed out its A BOY!! The doctor looked at me like I had rocks for brains, and asked me where I was, because she just had a GIRL!! I had seen the umbilical cord, and thought it was a boy. (Boy was I embarrassed!!!) Two of my sisters were outside of the room with my husband waiting, and they couldn't figure out what she had, because they heard it's a boy, and it's a girl. My husband, I could tell was a little disappointed, I think he felt that she was going to have a boy. But when my husband seen her gorgeous eyes looking up at him he was extremely happy with this beautiful child, and forgot all about wanting a boy.

After our last Grandchild was born (also a beautiful girl) my husband said he resigned himself to the fact that "We were in-capable of producing any male heirs"!! My daughter & her husband had known that she was a girl, but they didn't want us to be disappointed, so they never told us. As for me, as long as she was healthy that is all that mattered. But I reminded him, that it was the husbands who dropped the ball because they are the determining factor in the sex of the baby. Even though we really thought we wanted a

Grandson, I wouldn't give up any of my precious Granddaughters. I love you all lots **Chelsey, Christine, and Ashley!!** (Names changed to protect the innocent)

My husband's mother had also hoped for a Grandson herself, to carry on the family name. After we had two daughters, we waited too long to have another one, (I was on birth control-SHE NEVER KNEW).It was better for us, because I was a fertile myrtle, and we didn't want a kid every year! My husband's father was an only child, and his older brother never married. Our youngest daughter's husband took our family name, but they never had a Son. So the Shaffer name is going to die off with us.

Chapter 36

Yesterday, (Wednesday Feb 8) Karlyn and I were finally able to get together for lunch. We had a really wonderful time. She finally received the afghan I had made especially for her for Christmas. (Better late than never). She let me know all the things that were happening at work, and what was going on in her life. I really miss not being able to work. I loved my job, and all the people I worked with were great. It was fun to get up and go to work each day. I know the Company is going through some major changes, and it is really stressful for her, but hopefully it will settle down, and she will enjoy the job as much as I did. Most big companies are taking the personal service out of Customer Service, and I think it will be a big mistake for them. The Customer is supposed to be the top priority, and to not cater to the Customer any more is a BIG mistake!

She still looks fantastic. If she is under a lot of stress, it sure doesn't show!! She has been such a wonderful friend, I'm so glad we had the opportunity to work together for so many years. I really value the friendship that we formed. We had many, many laughs and heartaches over the years, but we were like the glue that held each other together.

I was on my way home from work one night, when a semi hit a bird and it flew into my car!! I had seen him hit it, and when I seen it heading for my car, I thought it was coming through the windshield!! But luckily it flew into my grill. I did not realize the damage it caused, until I got home and looked at the front of my car. It tore a huge hole in the grill (of course with these new cars being plastic, that wasn't hard to do) and the damage was going to cost $1200.00 to fix!!

Of course when the people at work found out what had damaged my car (Karlyn made sure everyone knew) I received a lot of teasing. The next day when we went to lunch, there was a rubber chicken strapped to the front of my car when we walked out the door. I laughed so hard, I thought I was going to wet my pants!! (Karlyn had gotten the rubber chicken from the poultry buyer.)

When I looked up, there were lots of people standing in the lunchroom windows just laughing hysterically. (At my expense)!! She never let me forget it after that. Each year since then, she gets me some kind of Chicken ornament to go on my tree, and I value each and every one of them!! (Needless to say, they are collector ornaments, so they are an expensive reminder!!)

She has done quite a few stunts at my expense, but I love her dearly, and my life would have been pretty dull without her! She also gave me a good luck doll. She bought it, because she said the legs reminded her of me, they are long, and pencil thin-LIKE MINE (everyone at work called me bird legs) (thanks to her), and she gave it to me for my surgery. I already told my family, that the doll cannot be in the operating room, but I expect to find it in my bed when I wake up from surgery! She is packed in my suitcase waiting to go. Karlyn, thank you for your special friendship!!

Chapter 37

A few weeks ago, I watched a show with Barbara Walters called "Where is Heaven?" She was interviewing people from all different religions backgrounds to get their view as to what, and where heaven is. I was really surprised to hear some of the answers. A lot of the answers that are different than my views really got me questioning my faith in what I thought I believed. Almost all of them believe that there is an extreme being, and that there will be a better place waiting for us when we leave our earthly bodies. Quite a few believed we are reincarnated again, when we are through living our life as we now know it.

Then there is the scientific facts that describe why people see what they do when they are dying that also made a lot of sense, and then there are the atheists that do not believe there is anything after this life, and when we die, we just die. I had never questioned the existence of God, and I truly believed there will be a better place to go to after this, but now I'm starting to question what I really think I believe!!

My belief has always been that there is definitely a God, and that there is a better place that we go to after we die, and that there is no such place as hell. I feel this way because when we loose a loved one, there is no greater pain in life that we have to endure. It is a living hell to go through, yet each of us has to go through this grief process many times in our lives, and still keep our faith in God. I could not bear the thought of ever loosing one of my children, or Grandchildren, yet many people have experienced this personal hell, and they must have had a strong faith in the fact that they were going to someplace better!!!

About a week after this, I had been shopping at Wal Mart, and they had the DVD collection of Oprah Winfrey's 20 years on T.V.I thought it would be very interesting to watch, so I bought it. It was a fantastic collection of some of her greatest shows, and I could not believe what she has done for so many people. She is such an amazing person, I have never cried so much from watching a talk show before. I E-mailed her to let her know what I thought of the CD's, but I didn't hear anything back of course (I never really expected to, but you never know). It actually helped re-new my faith in the fact that there is life after death, because there has to be some place better to go to.

There are too many bad things going on, that there has to be a better reward for all the people that unselfishly do good things for other people, and don't ask for anything in return.

Today is Friday Feb.10, my coordinator from the Transplant Center called and said that the three Antibiotics they put me on have been in my system for over a month now so they will be putting my name back on the Transplant list. Once again, she warned me to be ready because she really believes it will happen soon. I found out later, that I would have been called three times if I hadn't been taken off the list.

Chapter 38

Tomorrow is Saturday Feb.18, and it is my oldest daughter Bobbie Jo's 37th Birthday. She has asked for very simple requests. She wants to go out for a nice supper, and then on Sunday she wants me to make her favorite meal of pork chops, sauerkraut, and dumplings. I still haven't gone out and gotten her Birthday present yet, so I best get myself in gear. Her daughter Ashley's Birthday is Feb. 22, so I better get both presents while I am out.

Of course Ashley will be easy, because she loves Gift Cards. My daughter and her husband each share their Birthday month with one of their girls. Bobbie Jo shares it with Ashley, and Gary July 16, shares it with Chelsey July 21. I guess in a way that's good, because you get two done in one month.

Today is still Friday February 17, and I will try and tell you how my life was forever changed after this evening. For some reason, I could not fall asleep, so I grabbed my pillow and blanket and moved out to the couch to sleep, so I wouldn't keep my husband up also. It was a very cold evening (the coldest it has been in a long time) so since I have a leather couch, I went and got my electric blanket. It's now about 1:00 AM, and I'm finally warm and comfortable, and I fall asleep. At about 2:30, the phone rings and wakes me up. I look at the called ID, and it's from Life Source. At first I am too stunned to answer the phone because I feel it's just too soon, and my family still hasn't had time to get adjusted! But then I realize this is something I cannot survive without, so I pick up the phone. It is the transplant coordinator from Life Source, and she says they have a potential set of donor lungs. She tells me that I have two hours to get to the hospital.

We call our oldest daughter and Husband, and let them know what is going on. We tell them to take their time, because this could be a dry run. Our youngest daughter Kelly is already at our home, because she is getting a divorce from her husband, and is temporarily staying with us until she gets back on her feet again. We arrived at the hospital at about 4:45 A.M. I asked my family to hold off calling my siblings, because I wanted to make sure this wasn't a dry run. A very nice Doctor by the name of Dr. Black (my nickname for her) came in at about 8:30, and introduced herself to us, and said she was going to be the one going and retrieving the new lungs. She also explained in detail all about the surgery and all the risks involved with the surgery. She said I would be put on a heart/lung bypass machine (which is risky in itself) and I would have about five drainage tubes, and be hooked up to lots of monitors. Then she explained the risks, and the list was sooo long, I didn't want to think about that because I resigned myself to the fact that I was going to live and I didn't want to listen to all that could happen!!! It's a good thing it happened so fast, because you really can't possibly take in everything they tell you, or you would probably chicken out. So I signed agreeing to have the surgery. Then the nurse came in and said that I had to take a shower from head to toe with this antiseptic soap. So my daughter helped me accomplish this. After I finished the shower, if there was any doubt in my mind whether I needed the surgery or not, this confirmed it. I wouldn't survive long without it.

At about 10:00 AM the nurse came in and said they had a chance to look at the new lungs, and they looked great. They were just waiting for an available operating room to remove them. So my daughter started calling my siblings to let them know that it was a go. All my family started arriving at the hospital. They all looked about as nervous as I felt, but they were all trying to stay up beat and positive.

The actual realization does not set in until they bring you to the quiet room right before surgery. When they took me to the quiet room at about noon, I met Dr. Red (my nickname for her) who was the surgeon that was going to perform the operation, and then they let all my Family in to see me before they took me to the operating room. I was trying to be very strong for all of them then the realization hits you that you may never see them again, and no matter how hard you try you just cannot hold it together.

My siblings have been very supportive while I made my decision. We had gone through a similar experience with my mother with many, many set backs, that I felt really bad that they had to go through it all over again with me. We are very close to each other, and I could see the fear and pain in all their eyes!!! I love them all so very much, and I could feel their strength, prayers, their encouragement and their love being transferred to me. I kissed them all for luck, and then the tears flowed.

Saying good-bye to my Husband and Daughters was not quite so easy!!!!!! This was the hardest thing that I have ever had to endure in my life. I just wasn't ready for it, it wasn't because I was afraid I was going to die, I just wanted to hold on to them during the surgery and not let GO!!!! Of course that wasn't possible, so we had to say Good-bye. It was very heartbreaking and emotional, lots of crying I tried to radiate all the love I've ever had in my heart for all of them to them, Tom, Bobbie Jo, Kelly, Gary, and the Grandkids are my whole life. I like to harass my son-in-Law, but he is like a son to us.

My husband was the last to leave, then the reality set in, and I was very scared for the first time. He has always been my rock, and has always been there for me, but this was something I had to do alone, and I was on the verge of losing it entirely. When he hugged and kissed me, he told me I was going to be just fine and he would see me after surgery. I thanked him for all his love and support and all the wonderful years of marriage. Then he left, and I was all alone for the first time. They then brought me to the operating room. I prayed to God to keep me safe and that if it was my time to go, PLEASE, PLEASE, give me one more day. Today was my Daughter's birthday, and I didn't want her to associate her Birthday with the death of her mother. Also, her Grandma's Birthday was December 7th (Pearl Harbor) And mine is Sept 11 (Terrorist attack) so lets keep the rest normal. Then they put me to sleep.

Chapter 39

They told my family that the surgery would take about 6 or 7 hours. After I had been in surgery for about an hour, they heard a helicopter land on the roof of the hospital, and they all were excited because they figured it was my lungs. A little while later a nurse came out and said the lungs were good, and the operation was a go.

About 3 hours later a nurse came out again and said that they had taken out and replaced one lung, and they were starting to remove the other lung. Then after about 2 hours later, they said they had finished putting in the 2nd lung, and were starting to close. They told my family that they did not have to use a heart/ lung by pass machine because they took out the worst one first and that the other one was able to sustain me until the second lung was in. Dr. Red came out when she was done, and said that everything went very well, she said my new lungs are really nice and pink, but that my old lungs were really gross and in really bad shape.

They brought me right up to I.C.U. They let my family come in two at a time to see me. They all never realized how much stuff I would be hooked up to, and how bad I was going to look. It was kind of a shock to all of them but even my sister Colleen, who hates I.C.U came in to see me (I'm proud of her). From that night on, my husband and my oldest daughter Bobbie Jo both stayed at the hospital 24 hours a day while I was in I.C.U. Then when they moved me upstairs they took turns nightly sleeping in a recliner in my regular room so I wouldn't be alone. The first night of surgery, I guess I had a very bad night. My stats would not stabilize and my levels kept dropping off. Dr.

Black was at the hospital most of the night because she had a couple of us patients with problems.

The next day after my surgery Dr. Black came in and said that I had blood pools in my right lung, and that they had to take me back into surgery and re-open the right lung and get the blood pool out. Luckily they were able to go back into the same incision, so they didn't have to leave another scar.

A few days later they took out the respirator tube, and put me on oxygen which I tolerated very well, I was kept in I.C.U for a couple of days more, then I was moved upstairs to a regular room.

The first night I was moved out of ICU and put on a regular floor at about 4:00 A.M. the door opened, and 3 nurses and a doctor came into the room. They said I was having a heart attack, and didn't I feel all the pain? I told them that, I was always in a lot of pain since my surgery, and how would I know if I had any added pain!! They also had called a code blue for the gentleman in the next room, so running between his room and mine, they sure had double trouble!! They were giving me all kinds of stuff to bring my heart rate and blood pressure down. But because of having a Lung Transplant, some of the fluids they gave me were too much for me because then my oxygen level started dropping off and they called, for pulmonary stat!! I knew I was in trouble but the thought of not surviving the heart attack had never occurred to me, the only thing I was actually thinking about was that they said I could have a coke (which I had been thinking about for days,) when I was better at swallowing and now I was not going to get the coke I wanted. That sure was a dumb thing to be thinking about when I could have been dying. They finally called in the head cardiac Doctor, and he moved me back to ICU to get me stabilized again. I spent another four days in ICU. I however must have passed out, or they put me to sleep, because I don't remember the trip back to ICU, or what happened after that. I woke up the next day. Sometimes I guess not being aware of everything going on is a blessing in itself.

If you are a vain person, when you spend time in ICU, your vanity goes right out the window. You are seen from head to toe by so many doctors; you forget what each one does. The nursing staff in ICU is the greatest!! They are there to make sure YOU are well taken care of, and you are their only concern. They stay in the room with you, and they constantly check out everything so they can report any problems immediately to the Doctor. At first I was extremely embarrassed when I had two male nurses, but they were very caring people, and as long as they did their job and made me comfortable, it bothered me less and less. In fact, these two nurses actually ended up being my favorite.

After a few more days in intensive care, they were able to move me back upstairs. They started getting me up more and walking around, and I started going to Cardiac and Pulmonary therapy. They had me walking on a treadmill, and I had never done that before, so let me tell you my legs were mighty sore after the first day. Having my husband and daughter with me was a great inspiration to me; my husband even did the exercises with me in physical therapy. They never slacked off with me, when they thought I needed pushing, they pushed and if they thought I was over doing it, they told me to back off. My family was at the hospital quite a bit to see me. So I had a lot of company, which I was very grateful for. I never had a chance to get lonely. We even went upstairs to the Cafeteria for supper a few times. I had my surgery on February 18, and was finally let out of the hospital on March 7, along with half of the drugs in the pharmacy!!!

Chapter 40

I was very curious when I got home, as to what everyone was thinking the night I had my surgery. I know myself I was terrified, but I wanted to know how everyone else felt, so I asked everyone if they could write a paragraph and let me know what they were feeling the night of my surgery. Here are some of the feelings from my family:

Husband Tom:

I was not at all worried that you would not make it through the surgery. Because other than your bad lungs, the rest of your organs were in perfect shape. What I was most concerned about is that your system would reject the new lungs. I had already made up my mind weeks before the surgery, that the Transplant was a necessary operation for you to be able to live a normal life again, and a quality one. When we spent the week at the University they had given us the odds of survival, and I felt we should make an appointment with your lung specialist to get his opinion of going through with the transplant. He said it was your decision to make, but he wasn't a big supporter of the surgery, because he felt the odds of survival hadn't gotten any better than when they first started doing lung transplants. I asked him that if you decided not to have the surgery done, and with the condition of your lungs how could you handle another bad bacterial infection or pneumonia again like you had the previous year? He said that your lungs were on a down hill spiral, and that you probably would not survive another infection, so he suggested that we have a DNR put in your file. I made up my mind right then and there, that I was not willing to loose you yet. Having the surgery would give you a few good quality years, and that sure was better than none at all. When you got a chance to hug everyone before you were brought into surgery, I was the last one to be with you. You said good-bye to me, and I was upset with you for that. I wanted you to say to me, "see you when I wake up" but instead you said good-bye and thanked me for our wonderful life together. That was very emotionally upsetting to me, because I wasn't expecting you to say that. I really appreciated the fact that they kept coming out to give us updates. When they finally came out and said they were finished and closing you, I was able to breathe a heavy sigh of relief. I said to the family," We won the first major battle, and now we begin to fight the war on rejection".

My entire Love Forever, Tom

Daughter Bobbie Jo:

Let me start by saying Bridget Shaffer is not only my mother but my best friend. My name is Bobbie Jo and I am Bridget's oldest daughter. Originally when my mom asked me to write about what I was feeling the night of her surgery, I thought no problem I can do that easily. But the more I thought about writing my feelings down, the more worried I became as to how she would re-act to reading this.

My sister and my aunts and uncle were very positive that everything would be fine. I wish I could say I had that same feeling. The evening we got the call, my husband Gary and I had been over at a good friend's home, celebrating my birthday. I was feeling no pain when we arrived home later that evening from our friend's home. We went to bed around 12:30 a.m. A couple of hours later my dad phoned letting us know they were heading to the hospital. They received a call from Life Source informing her they had a possible donor match for her lung transplant.

We woke our oldest daughter Chelsey to let her know where we going. She was both nervous and excited. We left promising to call as soon as we had more information. Our youngest Ashley was still sleeping. She has a lot of fears for a 12 year old so we thought it would be better not to wake her. Even though I had way too much to drink that night, I felt eerily sober when we arrived at the hospital. It took hours for all of the tests and x-rays to come back and each minute felt like an eternity. All of my mom's sisters, her brother and his wife came as well as my cousin Gina and her husband Chris.

When the news came from Dr. Black that everything was a go, she explained the risks which took about a half hour as well as the benefits, which took around ten minutes. Mom was told she needed to take a shower and scrub with this special antiseptic from her head to toes. She wasn't comfortable with the nurse assisting her, so I did. When they came up to get her for the surgery, I remember my heart sinking. We all went down to the pre-op room and were able to wait with her while she was being prepped. When it was time for her to go in, we were instructed to say our goodbyes to her. They meant till after the surgery when she was awake, to me however, it was a forever goodbye. My dad, my sister my husband Gary and myself, waited while her sisters and brother finished.

I remember my knees feeling like they were going to give out. My sister went first and when she left, it was my husbands turn. I remember my mom telling him he was like a son to her. Then it was my turn. I was shaking from head to toe. I remember the hug vividly and not wanting to let go.

Unfortunately, I do not remember a lot of what she said to me other than saying she didn't think God would be so cruel as to take her on my birthday, and that she would love me always.

I left the pre-op room crying so hard I collapsed in my husband's arms. When my dad came out he ran into my sister and I. which he did not expect after he stood hugging us for a while he went directly into the bathroom without looking back. When we went into the waiting room, I remember feeling that everyone was staring at me. They all looked so strong and I guess I couldn't understand why they weren't as upset as I was. When dad came in the room, I remember my husband letting go and my dad holding me awhile longer till I quit crying.

When we heard the helicopter, I remember going out in the hall with everyone and looking for it We couldn't see it, but we knew it was here with my mom's new lungs. There seemed to be a feeling of relief from everyone. To me it was just getting started. I do not remember the specific times the nurse came out to report her progress to us, I do remember her letting us know that she did not need to be put on By-pass. At this point I knew she was fighting. I could start to see the light at the end of the tunnel rather than the light to take her away.

The next thing I remember was mom's surgeon coming out to tell us she had pulled through and was doing great. Her old lungs were absolutely gross, but the new ones were nice and pink, and best of all working perfectly!! I remember such a wave of relief! I couldn't have asked for a better Birthday present!

Dad and I spent the night in the waiting room, if you want to call it that, (and every night after so she wouldn't be by herself. We alternated nights. We laid there for about 2 hours before we decided it was time to go back in and check on mom. When we entered her room in the ICU, we found out she had developed a serious complication. A blood pool had formed in one of the lungs and they needed to take her back into the operating room, open her back up and drain it. I remember being absolutely numb when I called everyone to let them know she was going back in for another surgery. Everyone came right back down to be with us again. They said this surgery should only take about one and a half hours. Four hours later the nurse came out to let us know that everything was good and they were finally able to control the bleeding.

I will always be thankful for the donor for the generous gift of life and their family for supporting that decision. But I will also always be thankful to the wonderful Doctors and Nurses at the University of Minnesota for the extraordinary care they gave my mom. I especially want to thank my mom for having enough love and courage for her and us to go through with the transplant and for having such a positive attitude through the last several years. I am very proud of her! She is my role model, my mother and my best friend.

I love you mom!!!

Daughter Kelly:

"Kelly wake up……were taking your mom into the hospital." Ooh no what's wrong now was the first thing I thought when my dad woke me up at

2:30 in the morning on February 18. I assumed my mom was having trouble breathing again and we were going to Cambridge medical center. I walked up the stairs half asleep and found my mom in the bathroom getting ready to go. My reaction was confusion. I remember thinking why are we going in? She looked alright to me. I asked my mom, "What's wrong?" "Why do you need to go to the hospital?" She responded "the U of M called, they have a donor." My heart fell into my stomach. I was shocked they already had a donor. We knew this day would be coming but I really didn't think it was going to happen as fast as it did.

The car ride to the hospital was fairly quiet. I think we were all in shock that it was happening so soon. I recall thinking is this a dream? Is my mom really going to get her transplant today? I looked over at my daughter sitting in silence next to me. I couldn't help thinking what if my mom doesn't make it through this. What if she can never see her three granddaughter's graduate, walk down the aisle, and have beautiful babies of their own. I quickly told myself to get those bad thoughts out of my head and concentrate on the positive. Like my mom being able to take a full breath and not feel like she is being suffocated anymore. For her to be able to live her life like she deserves to, instead of being winded from completing even the smallest tasks. It was hard not to worry but I was happy we contacted the U of M and that this procedure could give her back her life.

When we finally arrived at the hospital we were surprised once again to discover the hospital didn't have a sole around. After walking around for what seemed like forever we finally found a male nurse who helped us find out where we were suppose to go. We assumed she would go in right away but they told us they still had to go get the lungs so the transplant would not happen until later in the day. This made me think of the person who had passed away, donated their organs and made it possible for my mom to receive the transplant. I said a prayer for them and their family. I wondered if the person was young, old, male, female and how they died. I then said a prayer for my mom to watch over her and prayed that the lungs would be in good condition.

Most of the family had shown up to the hospital. We were all sitting in my mom's room talking when the nurse finally announced it was time to go down to pre-op for the surgery. My mom then had the opportunity to visit with us and her siblings before going in. Her siblings seemed very upset and everyone was crying, especially Colleen who was hiding around the corner in tears. I was nervous on the way down and was talking in my head to all my relatives that had passed away and that may be listening in heaven to watch over my mom. They must have been listening because I remember feeling an overwhelming sense of warmth and extraordinary calm. I was surprised by this since I thought it was going to be a lot harder to basically say my goodbyes to my mom but instead I was almost comforted. I was told my mom was going to be just fine. It's hard to explain. I didn't hear voices or anything, but somehow I knew in my heart that everything was going to be fine.

I bent over kissed and hugged my mom and relayed the message from the angels that she was going to be alright. I told her I wish I could go through the procedure for her. Even though I knew it was going to be OK I still wanted to take on the burden for her so she wouldn't have to. She had been through enough over the years. We then stepped out so my dad could have some alone time with her. I do have to admit how lucky I am to have such great parents that truly and dearly care for each other and us. I am blessed to be so lucky. I stood in the hall waiting for my dad to come out. When he did you could see the concern in his face. My dad would give his life in a heartbeat if it would help my mom, she is his world.

We all filed into the waiting room, tears still in everyone's eyes and prepared ourselves for the long and nerve-racking wait ahead. As I sat there I had one regret running through my mind........why didn't I tell my mom how sorry I was for what I put her through in my youth. I was a pretty rotten teenager and now that I have one myself I finally realize how much heartache I put my parents through. As I sat there regretting not telling my mom I was sorry I remember looking over at my sister who was sound asleep thinking, how in the world can she sleep and then I thought boy I wish I could get some rest but I was not about to go to sleep until I knew my mom's transplant was done and that she was doing alright. As I was thinking this the same warm sense of calm came over me once again. With this came a rush of wonderful memories. I remember all of our long talks at the kitchen table. We would sit there for hours just talking about any and everything.

I remember the vacations we took up to Peaches and Wally's cabin in Spooner, Wisconsin. We used to get up at the crack of dawn because we were so excited to go swimming. We use to walk in the woods at night and try to scare each other. I remember when my Uncle Gary wrapped my cousin Randy in tin foil, gave him an axe, and sent him in the woods to scare all of us girls. My cousin Angela got so scared she wet her pants. All of us kids use to follow suit with my dad when he would wash his face with ice cold well water from the pump in the morning and we would yell "Good Morning World!!" Our family get together's were always fun.

For the Holidays my mom would sew us matching outfits so every family wore the same color and patterns. As I looked around at my mom siblings I thought about my Aunt Patty who was not able to be there because she was at another hospital with her husband Doug who was going through his own battle for his life. She was calling for updates through-out the day and we were getting updates on his condition as well. I asked the Angels if they could pay a visit to them as well.

The nurse then came out to tell us the first lung was in and was strong enough to support her so that she did not need the bypass while the other lung was transplanted. "Thank God" was all I could respond with. The doc said the new lungs looked pink and healthy. It was then I knew for a fact that my mom was going to make it through this. I already knew she was strong willed enough to make it through the recovery and would have all of our love and support through out to make it.

I don't know who was looking over my mom that day but I guarantee she was being watched over. Their presence was strong and wonderfully consoling. I know without a doubt there were Angel's with all of us that day. It's hard to put their presence into words others can understand. But all I can say is when they are there and you are open to listen, their existence is undeniable, serene and reassuring. God Bless them and I know they will continue to watch over my mom.

Love, Kelly Jo

Sister Colleen:

I do not like being in pre-op or ICU units. I would prefer just to stay in the background, and not have to deal with the situation. I had a bad experience with my mother when she was in ICU, and had just woken up after Surgery. I was standing very close to her bed, and all of a sudden she reached up and grabbed my shirt, and was practically pulling me down on top of her, and that was very traumatizing to me. I couldn't get close to the bed after that, I would stay far enough away, so that no one could do that to me again. I found out later from her, that all she was doing was trying to talk to me, but with the respirator tube in, she was afraid I couldn't hear her. But after that no matter why she had done it, it had already logged itself in my brain. When everyone was saying good luck to my sister and giving her kisses. She knew I was hiding around the corner, but she told me to get in there, and I did.

At first, I really didn't know how I was feeling about her having this surgery. I was neither worried, nor not worried. Then I saw our parents. I told my sister Linda that our parents were there with us, but that there was nothing to worry about because they were not here to take her with them, but they were here to watch over her during the surgery. That really put my mind at ease, and I was no longer worried about her not making it through the surgery.

I am a firm believer in God, and I also believe in Angels. I believe angels are all around us, and that each of us has a guardian Angel. When my sister was really sick and in ICU last year, both my sister Linda and I sent our own guardian angels to watch over her. After she was released from the hospital, she said that she knew she was not alone, because every once in a while a figure would walk across the hall, and stand there until she noticed it, then move on. It would never turn around so she didn't know if it was male or female, but she wasn't afraid of it either. Of course she said she never asked it who it was, because she wasn't THAT comfortable with it! So, I knew she would survive the surgery, and I'm looking forward to seeing her have a normal life for a while.

Love Colleen

Sister Linda:

By Linda: A documentary from my perspective of what took place on the day of Bridget's double lung transplant:

At approximately 8:30 AM on Saturday, February 18, I received a telephone call from my sister Mary informing me that Bridget was in the hospital since 1:30 AM in the morning. My first thought was that Bridget was back in the hospital because she was very sick again and my heart sank. Then Mary explained that Bridget was at the University of Minnesota waiting for a double lung transplant – my heart sank even further. Mary said that Bobbie Jo was going to call her back and that she would get back to me with additional information as soon as she knew more.

I could hardly get up and out of bed – I was moving so very slow – I could not move any faster. Mary called me back about half an hour later and said that Bridget may be going into surgery around 2:30 PM if everything is okay with the donor lungs. We decided to meet at Mary's house at 12:30 PM so that we could be at the hospital by 1:30 PM – Mary said that she would call Colleen and inform her of our plans. Colleen called me shortly thereafter and had asked if I would pick her up – I told her **"No"** (my thoughts were that something wasn't right) – I told Colleen to meet us at Mary's house at 12:30 PM instead.

As I sat on the couch sipping my coffee trying to grasp just what was happening, I became very frightened. I was second guessing my conversations with Bridget about having a lung transplant – what if Bridget does not make it? Because I took part in encouraging Bridget to have this lung transplant – I felt a heavy burden weighing on my shoulders. A thought kept coming to my mind, "Why didn't I write Bridget a letter back when she wrote me a letter explaining that she was going to go through with the lung transplant." I kept having this feeling that we were not going to make it to the hospital in time to see Bridget before her surgery and that we needed to get down to the hospital sooner. I called Mary back with a ***panic*** in my voice and told her that we should be down to the hospital no later than noon instead of 1:30 PM, and that I would meet Mary at her house by 11:00 AM. I told Mary that I would call Colleen and have her meet us at her house by 11:00 AM instead – Mary agreed right away. I called Colleen with a ***panic*** in my voice and repeated the same message as I gave to Mary – Colleen agreed right away. I was still feeling nervous and I knew that I had to move faster even though my feet felt like lead. **I knew of only one thing to do:** I ran up stairs so fast and I kneeled before my beautiful picture of Jesus I have hanging on the wall in my reading room…and then…

I prayed, and I prayed…I cried and I cried, "Oh please God let Bridget survive this lung transplant – let Bridget live. I then sat on the ottoman in the room and I felt God's presence and I knew God's peace was overflowing into me and I felt that God was saying ***"Bridget is going to be fine – you need to trust***

me – how many times have I told you that – my thoughts were with you when you discussed a lung transplant with Bridget and my thoughts were with you when you knew Bridget would have a lung transplant and when you knew that Bridget would speak later of her experiences months ago." I felt comfort and happy for Bridget, and I was able to get dressed in a hurry and I ran out of the house and drove to Mary's. I could not get Bridget and the surgery that she would be undertaking out of my mind – but they were happy thoughts. I reached Mary's house only to find that Colleen was not there yet. I became nervous again, my mind said that we have to hurry up and get to the hospital – we have to be there before Bridget goes into surgery, still thinking that surgery was not going to take place until 2:30 PM. I called Colleen's house and Frankie said that Colleen left about 45 minutes ago. I started to be concerned about Colleen driving to Mary's house – wondering if I made the right decision about not picking up Colleen – then I thought if she is not here soon, we will have to leave. Ten minutes later, Colleen arrived. We left Mary's house right away and headed straight to the hospital – ***we needed to be with our sister – we needed to hurry!***

When we arrived at the hospital and went to Bridget's room, she was still there and I was surprised at how calm I was and how calm Bridget seemed to be. I really did not know what to say…I don't think that I said much. We were not in Bridget's room long when we all had to go to the bathroom. Just when we were returning from the bathroom, they were taking Bridget down to surgery. It was ironic how we just made it in time and how we were able to go to the bathroom before walking Bridget down to the operating room. This short walk was tough, and with each step, it became harder. Once we were all in the pre-operating room with Bridget, I felt more at ease – I almost knew that Bridget was going to make it through – I almost felt certain. I hugged Bridget and said my "goodbye" (I am not sure what I said to Bridget, it felt rather odd, yet I knew that she was going to be okay…it was not really a goodbye…it just felt strange.) I thought it kind of odd that I did not feel like crying – Colleen and Mary were crying huddled in the corner. I felt strong, I called to them to say goodbye to Bridget – they automatically moved forward with strength and said their goodbyes to Bridget. We walked out of the pre-operating room and I felt that Bridget would be fine – why wasn't I frightened anymore? What happened to my emotions?

We were a picture of a blessed and beautiful family while waiting in the waiting room during Bridget's surgery. We were all together heart and soul. I found it hard to leave my seat – my butt felt glued to the couch – just a quick run down the hall to go to the bathroom from time-to-time and back again. I felt pain for Bobbie Jo, Tommy, and Kelly – what must they be going through – but I really wasn't focusing much on them, my thoughts were with Bridget. With all of us sitting together, it brought back memories of all of us waiting in the operating waiting room while Mom had her heart surgery. We bonded just like we did the evening of mom's heart surgery – we needed to be there for Bridget and for each other – <u>and we were!</u>

Bridget's coordinator came out to say that they opened up Bridget and they were ready for the lungs to arrive very soon (I did not like the fact that they opened Bridget up and that the lungs were not there yet). A half hour later, Bridget's lungs still hadn't arrived – I started to get uncomfortable again, even though I felt that Bridget was going to be fine. We waited longer and still no lungs…then, I heard the sound of a helicopter overhead that was landing on the roof of the hospital. Oh what beautiful music to my ears – joy sprung to my heart – I said "it's a helicopter" – I ran into the hall and looked up to see the helicopter but I could not see it…I felt excitement…I walked back into the waiting room. Someone said it was just a truck outside, but I knew it was the helicopter (Mary, Colleen, and Kelly heard the helicopter also) so we went back out into the hall to see if we could spot the helicopter, that's when Tommy's brother Gary arrived. Gary said that there was a helicopter landing just above and he looked for the helicopter with us. We went back into the waiting room. My excitement was building – a precious, precious double lung from another was going to be shared with Bridget to give her new life (I was not thinking about the donor and their family; I could only think about Bridget and her family.) The coordinator came back out to inform us that the lungs were here and they were putting them in Bridget. Oh what a joy!!

The hours ticked by, I said a lot of "Our Father's and Hail Mary's," silently and waited like everyone else. Finally, the doctors were standing on the other side of the door, and we all came fully alert – and after about a minute, which seemed like such a long time, the doctors came into the room. All eyes were focused on them as if trying to read their minds. We didn't have to, Dr. Red said that Bridget did well and that the lungs she had received were beautiful, they removed her icky lungs, and Bridget did not have to go on the bypass machine. We were thrilled – we were also very glad that it was over and that Bridget was doing well. We were told that in a half hour, they would be bringing Bridget up to the fourth floor intensive care unit and we could go up to the waiting room on the fourth floor. We all practically ran out of the room – we were hurrying up to the fourth floor right away to make sure that we would get there in half an hour. About two minutes later, we were in the fourth floor waiting room – Bridget was <u>not</u> there yet! What was taking so long – it felt like a half hour to us. We patiently waited, and then we un-patiently waited. We went into the hall to scope it out – where is Bridget? We were told a half hour and times up – our sister better get up here soon. Finally, we had enough, and after 45 minutes, we investigated – Bridget was in her room (they never told us) with the curtains half closed, they just brought her up from surgery. We were told that when they are done doing what they have to do, we could each see her for a few minutes – I took a peek into the room anyway just before I left – and yes, that was my sister Bridget lying on the bed with tubes everywhere (oh, I should not have peeked, I got a little scared of what I saw – I should have waited until they were done).

We were told that we could see Bridget – I don't remember, but I think I went with the first group and I also don't remember who I went with. I just remember they were <u>not</u> all done; they were still setting things up. The nurse said that Bridget was doing well – her color to me was a bit ash – but her vital signs looked good. I kept thinking, "How is Bridget going to feel when she wakes up and is on a respirator." Tears sprang to my eyes and I thought of all of the pain she is going to be in when she wakes up. After seeing mom and Gary on a respirator, we were all afraid of respirators. After a few minutes in Bridget's room (and a lot of questions later), I had to leave so that someone else could go in to see Bridget. I was okay with this because the nurses seemed very confident and they seemed to know what they were doing. I felt that Bridget was in good hands or God's hands so I left.

Colleen, Mary, and I left the hospital and we talked and talked all of the way home – we were exhausted but we felt good and things were going well – Mary and I would meet again tomorrow morning to see Bridget. When I returned home, I thanked God and I prayed for Bridget's recovery – I really felt that Bridget would be fine and that she was in God's hands – I needed to let go and to let God take over.

By Linda: A documentary from my perspective of what took place on the second post-lung transplant day of Bridget's double lung transplant:

Early the next morning, I received a telephone call from Mary that they had to take Bridget back into surgery. My first thought was "How could this happen, I felt so certain that Bridget was going to be fine" and then I thought, "How can Bridget survive another major surgery?" I was confused, I felt certain that God was saying that Bridget is going to be fine. I hurried to the hospital, but when I arrived, no one was in Bridget's room, so I ran down to the surgery waiting room and found everyone there. Tommy said that there were blood clots at the top of one of Bridget's lungs that is why they had to do another surgery – to flush out the lungs and to clean out the blood clots. We all were very quiet during this surgery even though we were told that it would not take that long – we were numb, we never expected this to happen. I was nervous and I had to go to the bathroom often (Bobbie Jo and Kelly Jo were going to the bathroom a lot as well).

After about two hours, we still did not hear anything, everyone started talking and we were all continually looking up at the board on the wall where they note when a patient is in the recovery room – Bridget was still in surgery. Every time a doctor would come out of the surgery room door, all eyes were focused on that doctor to see if it was Bridget's doctor – there were so many people in the waiting room and so many doctors that came out of the door. Every time that I went to the bathroom, I waited outside the post-surgery room, big double doors for a minute or two to see if I could see Bridget…there was no Bridget.

Finally, Bridget's doctor came out of the door and said that everything went well and they flushed her lungs to remove the clots – they thought the clots were from Bridget's body in her old lungs during the first surgery. We were told that they would be bringing her back up to the fourth floor intensive care unit in half an hour. We all felt okay – she made it through a second surgery and survived maybe she would be okay – Tommy said these things happen it's just a bump in the road.

We were all exhausted, and this time, we slowly walked up to the cafeteria to get a bite to eat. After we all ate (somewhat fast) we went to the fourth floor waiting room and were going to wait for Bridget there. I know that we were all thinking poor, poor Bridget, she had to endure another operation and I know we were all thinking her healing time will be longer because of everything that she went through.

At that moment, I felt Mom's presence and my spirits lifted. I asked Mary to go with me to the patient elevator doors on the fourth floor where patients return on a set of elevators after surgery. These were the same doors where we were all waiting for mom when she came back from heart surgery – the feeling felt the same to me. I started to get excited to see Bridget and I felt that I needed to see her and let her know that she is going to be fine even though she would be still under – I felt my soul somehow could touch her soul. Every time the doors would open, Mary and I stood very still and our eyes were glued on the elevators doors to see who they would be bringing out. No patients, just doctors, nurses, and hospital staff. Finally, our Bridget was coming through the elevator door, and as though I was in a trance, I walked beside Bridget as they were wheeling her down the hall and hand-pumping air into her lungs. My first thought that came to mind while I was walking next to Bridget was, "This is my sister Bridget and I am going to protect her in any way that I can, so I walked along with them to Bridget's room (the hospital staff never looked at me and I don't even know if they knew I was there). Once they wheeled Bridget in her room, I knew for now only that Bridget was okay. I went back to tell the others that Bridget is back in her room.

My thoughts were vague for the remainder of the day and the following day. On Wednesday, I went back to work and visited Bridget during the evenings after work. During Bridget's recovery, I don't remember much of who, when, what, and where, but I remember one evening soaking in the tub and crying my heart out to God – I wasn't so certain anymore and asked God, "If Bridget is not going to make it, please keep her alive so that she can breath normally with her new lungs for at least one day. After all that Bridget was going through, I pleaded with God to let her breathe." Things were up and down with Bridget, but after her heart attack, I felt things started to improve. I could see that things were improving with Bridget and we were able to walk around the floor of the hospital for a few days. Then the doctors thought that Bridget's system was entirely rejecting her lungs (I was not aware of this when I went to the hospital to see Bridget that evening after work). Bridget, Bobbie Jo, and Gary explained what happened to Bridget and said that she was <u>not</u> rejecting her lungs. Bridget looked great – instantly I knew once again that she would be fine – but there was something else going on. I cried and smiled all the way home. When I returned home, I called Colleen and said that, "Bridget had received a miracle." Colleen agreed with me that, "Bridget had received a miracle."

Conclusion:

I am learning to trust God more and more each day. If we listen, we will hear God's messages to us (we will not hear the spoken words out loud, we will hear them whispered in our mind and in our heart). For example, when Gary died, the heart rate machine showed a flat line, and instantly, I was told ***"Do not leave yet, there is going to be one more heartbeat."*** His brother Billy tried to get me to leave and I would not go, because I was waiting for one more heartbeat. I waited, and still there was a flat line on the machine, and I continued to look at the machine and to wait. At last, so ***delicate,*** so ***beautiful,*** and so ***small***, there was one more heartbeat and I knew that there is life after death for I was told to wait for this sign, which started me on the path of my spiritual quest and my search for God. The hardest thing for me to do is to trust God at times when I am afraid, even though I've been told more than once. Be open to God's words…He will send you his messengers, He will send you messages through people, books, and other sources, and He will send you whispers from your angels…for God is speaking to you…listen and trust…

What I know is that we can only be certain of the moment no one knows what tomorrow will bring – live each day with love in your heart and listen to the messages from God. For the moment, we are alive and Bridget is alive, and I know there is more meaning in Bridget's life than you realize…God has plans for Bridget and her journey is not done…and He has plans for you too…be not afraid…we are in God's hands…may His will be our will and may it be done:

Love, Linda

Brother John:

I have been asked by my sister to write a few words on the emotions I was feeling on the day of her lung transplant surgery. I remember it was a dark and stormy night---ooh wait a minute that is a different story!!

What I do recall when we received the news on that Saturday morning was having some apprehension as we were driving to the hospital. As the family started to arrive and we found out that the surgery would likely happen, I became more at ease. While we were in the pre-op room waiting with her before surgery I felt a confidence that all would go well with her surgery. I knew my sister had a strong will and had some of the best surgeons that you could want, but it was tough to look around the room and see the pained looks on some of our family member's faces. I wanted to console them but not contribute any tears of my own, (as a male you are always supposed to show strength in times of difficulty.)

I felt my sister needed to know she made the right decision about the surgery, and that we would see her again in this lifetime. I remember telling members of my family while we were waiting that she would do well and the surgery would be smooth sailing. That day ended well, the surgery went off with no complications. However-----the emergency surgery to soon follow is another story for another time.

Love You Bridget

Sister Mary:

This was a very hard thing for me to go through, because Bridget and I are very close. I was very worried and scared that she was going to have this surgery. But I knew that mom and dad would be watching over her. It was very emotionally draining to have to say good-bye in pre-op. I think all of us did a lot of praying to ourselves while we were in the surgery waiting room.

When the first person came out to give us an update she said that the lungs were there now, and they started the Transplant. It was a while before she came back out and told us that the first lung was in, and everything went well. It seemed like such a long time before they came back out again (we were all starting to get worried.) Finally the doctor came out and said both lungs were in, and everything looked great. When it was all over I was very relieved and happy. I couldn't imagine loosing my sister (favorite) and I thank God for allowing my parents to be there with us all.

Love Mary

Sister (out law) Jeanne:

Bridget, the day of your surgery I was thinking how nice it would have been to have been blessed with a sister like you growing up. I tried to make sure I let you know how much you mean to me. I also wanted you to know that if for some reason something didn't go right you could be at ease to know that John and I would always be there for your family. My thoughts were also thinking of the family of the donor who were grieving the loss of their loved one, but who had generously made the decision to give the gift of life so that others could live. Bridget, I'm truly happy you're a part of my life. I love you very much.

Your favorite sister Jeanne.

Son (Outlaw) Gary:

I am not sure why I have procrastinated so long on writing this, but here it goes. My name is Gary. Bridget is my mother in law. It has always been uncomfortable calling her my mother in law because she is much more than that to me. Bridget is my friend, mother to my wife, grandma to my kids, role model, and family patriarch and yes my mom.

I will never forget February 18, as long as I live. I have relived that day and those that follow many times. When Tom called to say they were heading to the hospital at 2:00 AM or so it changed many lives including my own.

As Bobbie Jo and I drove to the hospital, I initially was very scared that this could be the last time I see Bridget if the operation were not successful. But as I thought about all of the possible outcomes of the surgery through my head of what might happen this day, a sense of peace came over me. I realized that I had prayed for so often that this day would come that now that is was here it was in God's hands. I now started to think of how nice it will be to have Bridget with us for many years to come. I started to think about what it would take to get Bridget through this operation and how I could help her get stronger over the next few months to follow.

When we arrived at the hospital I began to watch how everyone was doing. Tom like always was stoic but I could tell he was also pre-occupied with the situation. My wife Bobbie Jo was doing what she did when she was nervous which transformed into doing everything she could for her mom to make her comfortable and help prepare her for surgery. I was really amazed at how calm Bridget was when I first saw her. I thought about how I would react if it were me with my family surrounding me waiting to hear if the surgery was going to happen.

Later in the morning more family started to arrive at the hospital. I was grateful to have several hours throughout the early morning with just immediate family present and was nervous for Bridget that the additional family may get too emotional for her. Again, she amazed me in how strong she was putting everyone at ease. Also, any doubts I had regarding the surgery were laid to rest in watching her get ready for surgery. Even the easiest of tasks were difficult. The reality of the situation was that without this surgery Bridget would not have long to live.

Saying goodbye at the surgery waiting room was one of the most difficult things I have done. I have only done this one other time when my step father Earl had heart surgery. I remember the emotion of watching my mother say goodbye to him just before the surgery. Those thoughts came back as I readied to say goodbye. I will never forget the words Bridget said to me. To summarize, she said she could not have asked for a better son in law. In truth, I could not have imagined a life not knowing Bridget.

In the week that followed the surgery I kept trying to think of how we could help Bridget get better. The whole week Tom and Bobbie Jo did not leave the hospital except to shower and get a change of clothes. Bobbie Jo and I talked about Bridget and Tom getting an apartment at the U of M. I suggested to Bobbie Jo that she talk to her parents about staying with us. My thought was that Bobbie Jo would spend a lot of her time with her mom during there stay at the U of M that could last a few months. I selfishly thought that I would rather have my wife here with me and the kids with Bridget and Tom. That way all of us would be together helping each other through this period of rehab. It turned out to be one of the best things that happened to us. The kids really enjoyed the opportunity to spend a lot of time with grandma seeing her get better than they have ever remembered her being prior to the surgery.

The surgery changed my life in a way I can't fully explain. I have a greater understanding of the power of prayer and positive thinking. I am at peace that no matter what happens after the surgery Bridget never gave up. She did everything she could to live and make a difference in our lives. I believe that this is a life lesson everyone needs to see. I also am thankful for the outcome for 2 people in my life. Tom and Bridget belong together. I could not imagine one without the other. Bobbie Jo lovers her mother so much and is so close to her. I was afraid for her if Bridget had not gotten this opportunity for the transplant. Finally, to the family of the lung donor, words can not describe how thankful we are for getting these lungs. Just know they went to a very special person.

Love Gary

Here is part of an article called "Attitude" written by Charles Swindoll which describes how I felt about this surgery:

"The longer I live, the more I realize the impact of attitude on life. Attitude to me is more important than facts. It is more important than the past, than education, than money, than circumstances, than failures, than successes, than what other people say or do. The remarkable thing is we have a choice every day regarding the attitude we will embrace for that day. We cannot change our past, we cannot change the inevitable. I am convinced that life is 10% what happens to me and 90% how I react to it"!!!

I tried very hard to go into surgery with a very positive attitude. I knew I wanted and needed this surgery, and even though the whole idea of it was terrifying to me, I am in charge of my life and what happens, and I knew without this surgery I didn't have much time left. But when you love life, it is very hard to embrace the fact that your life may soon be over. Now with the grace of God, and my donor, I can get a few more good years to spend with my family and siblings.

Chapter 41

When I left the hospital, my husband and I went and stayed at our daughter Bobbie Jo and her husband Gary's home. She lives closer to the hospital and we knew we had to go back and forth to the hospital a few days a week. We could have rented an apartment on campus for a couple months, but with my husband having to take a leave of absence with no pay, $1200.00 a month besides our home Mortgage payment would have been quite a bit more with less money. It has been just wonderful staying here. Between them and my husband, they are making sure I'm not doing anything I shouldn't be doing, that I'm eating properly and exercising. I am going to physical therapy twice a week and they are making sure I'm doing some type of exercise the other days.

They said it will take about six months for my chest to heal, and my new lungs to work up to their full potential. The ribs at the top of my chest are still really sore, but hopefully the pain should improve soon. I still have a couple infections going on with my new lungs, but hopefully they will start to disappear soon. They said that even though the infection may clear up in a few months, I still will have to take the Antibiotics for 12 to 18 months! (Oh good, I guess I'll be spending a lot of time in the ladies room!)

It was a wonderful time to be at the kids' home. I was very spoiled and well taken care of. We had a nice meal every night, and my daughter even did our laundry. Even though I wasn't much company for them because I was recovering, even the girls came right in the room to see how I was doing as soon as they arrived home from school. We are a very close knit family, and we got even closer after this. I didn't ever think that could be possible but it happened. Our eldest Granddaughter had to give up her room for us, and she never once complained. The only time that it ever bothered me to stay with them, is one evening my blood pressure really shot up and they had to call the Transplant Co-coordinator to see if they should bring me in they said to increase a certain medication, and keep checking it they said if the bottom number went over 100 (it was at 96) to bring me right to emergency. It did not go over 100, but when I seen the look on my children, and grandchildren's faces they all looked scared to death, and it bothered me that what if I had a serious complication that I did not survive how bad would it be on them with it happening in their house? I said a prayer to God that if something was to happen please make sure I wasn't there with my Grandchildren.

Chapter 42

My husband is retired Military (Army). He spent 24 years in the Military doing many different positions during that time. He first served in the combat engineers as an anti-mine warfare demolitions specialist. He served in the Army Security Agency as a fixed station controller. To get back to our home state, he went into recruiting (Earning him a Recruiter of the year Award).

He also worked as a guidance Counselor for recruiting. He then went to work for the "Join Team", teaching & installing computers in the Recruiting Stations around the United States. And the last position he held before his retirement, he worked for the 88TH ARCOM as the (NCOIC) of Information Management. They covered a five state area installing computers, and fielding problems with their computers. He earned a **"Meritorious Service Medal"** for the job he performed. (This is one of the highest non-war time Medal that you can receive). He is very proud of this. He served in Vietnam twice. The first time was in 1965 (For 6 months) as an advisor. Then he served again in 1972 (for a year) as a demolition and mechanical ambush region 1 with the 101ST Division. When we found out that he was going back to Vietnam for the second time, we also found out that I was pregnant with our second child. We were both happy about the pregnancy, but in my mind there was always the thought of what if he doesn't come back? But with the help of God, he did come back, and was able to meet his second daughter.

He had taken a 45 day leave, so he could spend Christmas with us before he left to go to his next duty assignment (Okinawa).That year was actually the last year we ever had a REAL Christmas tree. He and his brother went out to pick out the tree, and they bought home the biggest tree that I had ever seen, it took up a full corner of the living room. However, by the time the holidays ended, when they took the tree down, they did not wrap it in anything, so needless to say by the time they got it out of the house, there wasn't a needle left on it!! I was vacuuming up tree needles after that for months, and believe me every time I vacuumed the house a LOT of cursing went on (addressed to HIM). I couldn't even put the baby down on a blanket, because I was afraid she'd find a needle!!

Tom left for Okinawa in January. Because he had been on a hardship tour just coming back from Vietnam the girls and I would be able to join him. We just had to wait for housing to be available, but his year in Vietnam counted as a year on the waiting list, so we only had to wait a couple of months before we were notified that we would be leaving June 3. (That is my brother's birthday). His assignment in Okinawa was a fixed Station Controller with the Army Security Agency. The military came in and packed us up in March, and the girls and I went and stayed with Tom's mom. Our furniture left months before we did, because it had to go by boat. I was very excited about being able to go and be with my husband but the thought of being away from my family was very hard to imagine. We all live in the same state, and see each other often. We are a very close family. I knew because of the cost, I just couldn't pick up the phone and call them whenever I needed someone to talk to, so I'd have to rely on letters. We could use Ham radio (which I did a few times), but it's not very personal. I tried to send as many pictures as I could, so they could watch the girls grow up.

My biggest problem is that I am terrified to fly!!! (I still am). I think the biggest reason is that I want to be in control of my life, and I have to rely on someone else, and there is a lot of people I won't even drive with, because they are lousy drivers!! Also, it was a very long flight (12 hours).From here we had to fly to California, then to Hawaii, then to Guam, and finally to Okinawa. My Doctor suggested that I take a valium to calm my nerves, but with two daughters one not even a year yet, and the other one 3 ½ years, that would have been all they needed a SPACE CADET for a mother!! So, I passed on the pills.

The day before we were scheduled to leave, his mother and I went shopping for a new outfit, and we went to the beauty shop to get myself all spruced up for seeing my husband. I must say without being vain, that I really looked nice. My hair was very long, so I had it all put up in what was called Love Locks on top my head, and I bought a two piece outfit that consisted of a white pleated skirt, and a sleeveless blue blazer. We went by Pam Am, which was what they called a Mac flight. The Military used to charter commercial airline planes, and fill them with servicemen, and dependents. The flight went fine from here to California. But after that, it turned into a nightmare!!

We took off from California to Hawaii (after a short delay), and my youngest daughter started to scream her head off about three minutes after we were in the air. No matter what I did, I could not get her to stop crying. So many of the servicemen were so nice, they passed her around with a lot of them trying to calm her down. But, she wasn't about to be silenced, so they gave her back to me, and all I could do was wait until we landed to try and figure what was wrong. The steward came back and took my oldest daughter up front with him, to try and occupy her, because he figured I had my hands full already. He also told me that they made arrangements to have a Doctor waiting. When we finally landed, an ambulance crew boarded the plane and took me and the girls off the plane. They loaded us in an Ambulance, and drove to a spot next to the terminals, so they could examine her. The doctor said that the reason she was so miserable, is because she was starting to get an ear infection and that her ears hadn't popped (Even though I made sure she was sucking on her bottle) and that was causing a lot of pain and pressure. They wanted me to stay the night in a hotel, and wait to continue on the next day, but I told them I was too afraid to stay myself with two young daughters. I told them that as long as it wasn't life threatening I was getting back on that plane. He agreed with it, as long as we took her to the hospital as soon as we landed on Okinawa. He then gave her a shot of penicillin, and he pulled out a very small vial of something. He opened it up, and put two drops on her tongue, and within minutes she was fast asleep. He said that should make her sleep all the way there, but if she should wake up, only put one drop on her tongue and it should put her right back to sleep. I didn't know what it was, but I was sure glad I had it!!

In those days, you could smoke on air planes, and I really needed a cigarette by then. I did not notice that my oldest daughter had picked up the cigarette out of the ashtray, and then got scared to try it, so she was in the process of putting it back, when she dropped it in my lap. She was too frightened to say anything, so she said nothing to me about it. After probably a couple of minutes, I started to smell something burning, and realized it was me on fire. The GI sitting directly across from me also smelled it, and seen the smoke, so he jumped up and took the baby from me, and I was able to put the fire out with the can of coke I had!! I was too upset to scold her then, but I planned on having a talk with her when I calmed down. But it was actually my fault for lighting it, because obviously I didn't really want it, because it stayed in the ashtray most of the time until I put it out.

So, by the time we arrived in Okinawa my idea of surprising my husband was a total FLOP!! I looked like a physical wreck when I stepped off the plane. My hair was all falling down and in my face, my make up was all smeared, I had a couple runs in my nylons, and I had this huge stained hole in my skirt! My husband just stood there with this shocked look on his face, and said "What Happened?" The lady behind me said to him "Your wife deserves a medal for what she has been through! " I told him we needed to take the baby right to the hospital, and that I was too exhausted to explain what happened, but we'd talk about it after I had a long NAP. Then we went to the hospital, and the first thing they did was ask me for the Vial back. Reluctantly, I did give it back.

We were stationed in Okinawa for 4 ½ years and I'm pretty sure you don't want to hear everything, so I will give you the ones that happened, that has never happened before. (At least not to me)!!

When our belongings finally arrived and they delivered them, I told everyone not to wear the clothes in boxes, until I had a chance to wash them all, because they spent months on the ocean and needed to be re-cleaned again. Each cement double bungalow had a washer and dryer, but they also had a patio out back with a lot of clotheslines, and I love the smell of clothes after they have been hanging outside all day. The first load I found of clothes was my personal belongings. When I went outside to get them, I found out that every pair of my underwear were missing. Even the ones that matched the nightgowns! I soon found out why someone would steal underwear. The Government decided to order more men's stuff because they forgot about us wives. So I had to put in an order to Sears, and have them mailed to me. I wonder what they thought when they seen that order coming through? So for a couple weeks, until I received my Sears order, I had to wear my husband's underwear!! And the only thing I could think of was,"GOD please don't let me get into an accident with my husband's underwear on." My husband thought this whole thing was really funny. I told him that if the situation was reversed and he had to wear my bikini underwear for a few weeks, he also would have been extremely embarrassed. But then I pictured him in my underwear, and I sat and laughed for quite a while.

When we were there, we seen more of Okinawa, than we have ever seen of Minnesota, and we lived here most of our lives. For some reason, when people go somewhere temporary they make sure they see most of the places they recommend you to see. But there are a lot of people here that have never even heard of places that they (the tourist) found very interesting.

In Okinawa, they have Monsoon season (which is the rainy season) and this weather could cause a Typhoon. The Government then moves us to a Caution 4 which means an alert has been issued. You can always tell the new people there (we started calling them newbie's) they would run up to the PX and stock up on as much food as they could. (This was the first thing we did as newbie's also)!! Then the government would send us to caution 3 this meant the threat was more realistic. Then you'd start taking apart everything that wasn't nailed down that could blow away. After we got to caution 2, the "All Clear" was usually given, because the Typhoon took a different path. It was really scary at first but then you just got sick of them. After the first couple small ones came through, we learned it's best to have a few friends stay together.

The last Typhoon that came through in 1973 was a super Typhoon. We had three couples staying at our house with all the kids. You had to shove towels under the door, and under the windows to try to keep the water out. Since there was no power during these, you had to boil a gallon of water with a tablespoon of bleach to purify it. The kids were scared because of all the winds and rain, but as soon as they found something else to do they forgot the rain again. We sat and played cards in between eating and sleeping. We were finishing up a card game, when one of the kids came up and said that the kid's toys were floating on the screen porch. Of course we had to get up and look to try and figure out how this happened. Okinawa had big water roaches, and the first time I took our youngest out to sit on a blanket it was covered with these bugs! **GROSS**!! So when I laid her down for a nap, I went and investigated the screen porch, and seen one of these bugs crawling through one of these many holes. So I had this idea of filling all these holes with caulk. So I grabbed the caulking gun and caulk and finished filling all the holes! Tom and the other guys went out there, and all of a sudden he yelled for me, (I knew right then and there what I had done.) He asked me why I would caulk up all the drainage holes that let the water out. I told him I didn't think of the water, I just didn't want those bugs near my baby!!! They tried to take out some of the caulk, but I had packed too much in there. We ended up putting aluminum sheets on the roof and sides, so that when it did rain the water couldn't get in. (Another one of my bright ideas)!

The biggest excitement for the girls while we were on Okinawa is when Dad took mom for her driving lesson. I already knew how to drive an automatic, but my husband bought a Mazda which was a stick shift, and I had never driven one. He would take us to this remote road that ran along side of the airport, because it had a hill, and it was mainly used during the day. He told me that once I learned how to balance a car on an incline just using my clutch and gas pedal, (no brake) I could easily handle any stick shift. Our first lesson the kids had a great time. By the time I got the hang of shifting it into gear the car was already half way back down the hill. They would laugh and clap their hands and yell "DO THAT AGAIN MOM!!" and of course I obliged them for another month before I got the hang of doing it. When I finally did learn control, the girls didn't like it because; we didn't go backwards fast anymore.

We did have a fun time when we were Okinawa, but the greatest treat, was when we got off the plane in Minnesota, and seen our family waiting for us. It's nice to get away for a while, but it's even greater to get back home again.

Chapter 43

Having a Transplant is a very eye opening experience. You do it because when it's your only choice left the decision is easier to make for yourself. The year before was a very bad year for me, I was hospitalized five times. When they took out the respirator a few days after the second Transplant surgery, it isn't like instantly you can breathe. It just doesn't happen that way. (At least for me it didn't). You have to build up and train your new lungs to work properly. You go to physical Therapy when you have some strength built up and it really helps to re-build your large muscles. It wears you out, but strengthens you. After your Transplant, you have a lot of medicines to take, and you see their doctors quite often.

The U does an excellent job in taking good care of you. At first, after you are released from the hospital you go see the doctor twice a week. One good thing, is you get to see most of the patients that had their transplants at the same time as you did, and you get to swap stories as to how good it is going for them, and what set backs (if any) they have experienced. MY opinion of a transplant is that it is your last hope to be healthier, live a while longer, and once again have the ability to breathe. It's almost like a woman having a BABY. When you are in the hard labor stage, you hate your husband for doing this to you; all you want is it to be over with! But when everything is finally done, and you see the end result you forget all the pain, you no longer hate your husband, and you've been re-born to a higher purpose for your life.

Chapter 44

These past couples of weeks haven't been the greatest. No really major set-backs (In Health) but a few "tumbles" in the road. After one of my physical therapy sessions, I came home really sore) in my sternum and by the next day it had quite a large area that was black and blue. They made me an appointment with the transplant surgeon to take a look at it, and to see what could be wrong. They said it was probably just a loose wire, but they said I was to discontinue my therapy until she said it was o.k. to continue. We set up the appointment for Friday, and she was called in for a lung transplant about 10 minutes before I got there, so they re-scheduled it for the following Friday. The surgeon said the bone was like a step ladder, but it wasn't moving a lot, so it was best just to leave it alone for now. She said once they took the wire out, they couldn't reset another one in there, so unless the wire comes through the skin, they don't want to take it out. I was happy, because the other doctor said it was not a same day surgery, so I would have to be a guest of theirs for a few days. I told him no offense, but I'd prefer not to be a guest of theirs for quite a while.

Chapter 45

On Monday May 15, I drove to the hospital to have my lab work done, for the Transplant doctor that would be seeing me on Thursday, May 18. I had awoken up feeling fine, so I told my husband that I'd just take myself to the Hospital because all I was having done was labs. Plus, I have been going on short trips to the store and shopping to make sure that I was feeling alright to drive. The Doctor said I could if the medicine wasn't making me dizzy, and I am not having that reaction from any of the meds I'm taking.

Well, obviously, I wasn't as great as I thought I was. I really can't remember everything that went down, but I was on I35 heading home between Stacy and North Branch. Somehow I had veered too far to the right and found myself on the shoulder and I could not get the traction to get off. I finally got my tires to grab, and I turned the wheel as far as I could to the right. I had turned too much, and found myself heading to the center medium between me and the on-coming traffic. Before my tires could get into the ditch, I (really over compensated) turned the wheel again really hard to the right. The car started to slide and rotate on me then I lost control and she rolled twice, and I ended up upside down in the ditch.

The first Angel to arrive at my vehicle was an off duty EMT that was on his way back from Duluth. He did an excellent job at keeping me calm. I think I was so much in shock that I didn't realize how bad it could have been. A couple of other gentlemen started appearing with extinguishers and tools to try and help. I was still trapped in my seatbelt hanging upside down. I was terrified, but I remained very calm. He kept asking me questions to keep my mind busy. They could not get the seatbelt UN hooked, so they were going to cut the strap, but they didn't want me lying in all that glass that was beneath me, plus they didn't want to risk neck or back injuries. They were waiting for the paramedics to show up with a backboard. I told him that the pressure from the seatbelt across my neck and chest was really getting sore and was starting to really constrict my breathing. He knew by reading my medical alert bracelet that it had been less than three months since my transplant. They decided to try and get me out of my seatbelt.

The first attempt did not work they couldn't get the belt unclipped. So then they decided to use a knife and cut it, but the EMT said no. He had me check both my legs to see if I could move them and when he found out that they both were alright; they had me position my legs to take some of the weight off the belt. The other man climbed into the car and held one side of me up while trying to unclip the belt. While the EMT held up the other side of me. They were finally able to disengage the belt, and then they gently laid me on the floor. The EMT kept his head in the window at all times, so he kept talking and encouraging me as what they were doing.

The highway patrol and the firemen arrived first. Then the ambulance got there. They put a neck brace on me, and hauled me out the driver's window and onto a backboard. The good Samaritans helped them load me into the ambulance, and then they were gone. I was more upset that I didn't get to thank them, before they hauled me off to the hospital. The EMT with his encouragement and calming voice was able to make a very hard situation a lot easier to tolerate.

When I arrived at the hospital, the Doctor examined me, and wanted to know where I hurt the most? I told him that I wasn't in a lot of pain. My hip was sore from hitting it on the door handle, and my chest hurt from the constriction of the seatbelt, but other than a few cuts and bruises, I felt fine. They did a chest x-ray, a pelvic x-ray, and a hip x-ray which all turned out negative.

The doctor said I must have had an angel sitting on my shoulder to have been in a roll over like that, and have no major injuries. I told him I know I had two angels sitting on my shoulders. The first was the off duty EMT that happened to come by at the right time. And the second was my mother. Today is her Birthday, and she didn't want her Birthday shared with anything bad happening to one of her children. We haven't had too good of luck with normal birthdays. My birthday is September 11th; my mother-In Law's birthday is December7th, and now my accident on May 15, (mom's Birthday). At least this was a good outcome.

I called both my sisters Colleen, and Linda to let them know it was time now to call their Guardian angels home, because I couldn't seem to take very good care of them, and if they didn't take them back soon. I was probably going to kill them. Keeping an eye on me is like watching a bull in a China shop!!

I had an appointment on May 17, with my Transplant Dr. and he had another chest x-ray done to be sure that none of the rib cage was disturbed, and he said it looked alright. But since it was bruised quite a bit, it would probably take a while to heal. He also took my driving privileges away because he thinks I might have fallen asleep. So until they thoroughly check everything out, he won't let me drive. But he doesn't have to worry about that, because the Insurance Co. totaled my car, so unless I ride the lawn tractor, I don't have any way to get around. When you have a car and can go anywhere you never seem to mind if you stay at home all the time. But when you cannot drive, it dives you absolutely crazy to sit around the house all day. Luckily, my sister Colleen lives by me so she had no problem picking me up when I needed to get out. It also meant that one of my family had to drive me to the hospital all the time, and I didn't like that because they always narced on me to my doctor.

Chapter 46

Today is July 12, and I can't believe that I haven't written in my Journal since my car accident in May. It's not like I'm extremely busy or anything!! But after my accident I went into a depression I couldn't get myself out of. I don't know why I was so depressed, because I was happy to be alive. But for some reason I was also very deeply depressed. It took me a couple of months to get myself out of it. I'm better now. But I still have my bad days. (But who doesn't). It is very hard to be at home day in and day out. I look forward to my husband coming home from work and me going with him to the grocery store. (And I used to HATE having to go grocery shopping)!! As you can tell, it has been a very long two months, I'm going stir crazy. I am healing very well but it sure is a slow process. I'm still having lots of problems with the antibiotics but they keep switching prescriptions and doses to try and find something that agrees with my system. But, unfortunately it is starting to affect my kidneys also. But I'm sure once they get my system to agree with the pills, my kidneys will start to function better. So far the last two drugs have been working better together. It hasn't cured the problem yet but it is tolerable. I go back and see him on July 17, so I hope the tests show that things are getting better.

Chapter 47

My dad would always take it upon himself to help my mom around the house whether she wanted his help or not!! One day my older sister Colleen and I were getting off the school bus, and we seen my dad sitting on the upstairs window sill washing the outside window when all of a sudden he fell backwards out the window!! We ran home as fast as we could so we could see how he was. He was shaken up, but he said he wasn't in a lot of pain anywhere. He was very lucky that he didn't break anything because he landed on his back. My mom came running out the door, and we asked her what happened? She said that she was holding his feet to secure him, and the phone rang. Out of habit, she let go of him and went to answer the phone. She realized what she had done as she was leaving the room and ran to the window and seen him lying on the ground!! She thought she had killed him!!! I told her that before he completely recuperates she had better find a place to hide so he doesn't kill her.

Another time he thought he'd be nice and help with the laundry. We did not own an automatic washer (we had a ringer washer) and clothes were either hung on the lines downstairs, or outside (depending on the season). Of course I had a couple of my good mohair sweaters sitting on my bed that day, and he took them also to wash. He used hot water, and put my sweaters through the wringer. When I came home from school he said I was going to be really mad at him. I asked him what he did, and he said "come downstairs and I'll show you." He must have put the body of the sweater through first, and then pulled the arms through. The body of the sweater shrunk up to infant size, but the arms were at least three feet long!! It was so funny to see I couldn't stop laughing long enough to scold him for what he did. I did tell him later, that he was NEVER to wash another thing of mine!!! But did he listen?? NO he did not.

After my first daughter was born I spent a couple of months staying with my parents. Once again, he thought he'd be helpful and wash diapers for me. At that time we had cloth diapers and rubber pants. YES, he put all the rubber pants through the wringer, and popped holes in most of them.

Of course we kids were just as bad as dad with trying to help mom out. We liked to re-arrange the rooms and make fudge when mom and dad left for an evening. Of course we were given instructions before they left that we were not to re-arrange any room, and no making fudge!

As soon as they closed the door, the fudge pot would come out. Sometimes it turned out, but a lot of times we had to eat it with a spoon, or we stirred it too much and it was hard and sugary! We loved it anyway, no matter how it turned out. As we were eating the fudge, we'd decide which room we were going to change around that night. The next day we always got yelled at (or I should say I got yelled at because I was in charge) but she must have liked what we did, because she kept it that way until the next time we decided to re-arrange it again. My mother was very much a clean freak. You could eat off her floors. I don't know how she managed to do everything with six kids; we were not allowed to have a pet, because she thought animals were filthy. We also weren't allowed to spend the night at our friend's house, because she was afraid we'd pick up some kind of bug. But I guess it was alright, because we grew up fine without pets, and we never had bugs!! And believe it or not, most of us ended up quite normal!

Chapter 48

Today is July 17. I had an appointment with my lung Transplant Doctor. It was the monthly visit. I have to have blood work done, a chest x-ray, a pulmonary function test, (this test is to see how well your lungs age functioning) and then I see the Doctor. He checks me out and then goes over all the tests and blood work to let me know how everything looks, or if he sees something that is a concern to him. He took me off a couple of medications that I was on for a fungal infection in my lungs. But then he said that my blood pressure has been running a little higher than he would like it so he put me on a blood pressure medicine. (You loose some, you gain some!!) My chest X-ray showed a cloudy spot that has grown in size from the last chest X-ray, so he wanted me to have a CT scan done without the dye (because the dye is really hard on your kidneys, and so is a lot of the medicines I'm on). So we had to wait until they had time to fit me in. It turned out that it was just fluid on the outside of my lung. He thinks it was because my chest was bruised in the accident, I had some bleeding from the bruising.

Or, I told him that it might have been something really stupid that I did that irritated the bruising that was already there. I was in the garage trying to put something away that belonged on the top shelf. I was using a stool that had wheels. (That was really stupid, since we have four different size ladders that are all stacked up on the wall next to the shelves). YOU GUESSED IT, the stool started to roll out from under me, and I tried to grab on to one of the shelves for support. I put five long scratches on my arm from the metal shelves, a huge bruise on my arm, and of course on the way down, I hit the same bruise on my chest, and made it twice as big!! (Sometimes I don't use the brains that God has given me)!

After the Doctor stopped laughing (FIVE MINUTES LATER)! He went on to explain to me that because of the prednisone, I really have to be careful because I can easily break a hip, leg, or an arm, and I bruise more easier now because it makes your skin age and become transparent. (Boy he sure is right there, the front of my legs are a solid mass of bruises, it looks like a child's legs who is just learning how to walk).So he said I have to be very careful and think before I do something. I guess that was his way of saying "Stop doing stupid things!" For the time being they are just going to keep an eye on the fluid, and if it doesn't decrease they will have to do another CT scan, then decide what they will do about it. It doesn't bother me, and they don't seem concerned about it so I guess it's nothing I should be concerned about. That day ended up being very long. My first appointment was at 10:45, and we didn't leave the hospital until a little after 4:30 P.M. I for one am really glad that they re so thorough, and that all the doctors and staff really do care about you. But I really like Dr. D he has been my doctor from the beginning and he has always been so supportive. Your lungs are not only your own, but they are his also.

The next day, I had a mammogram scheduled at the hospital in Cambridge. (This is where I usually go).This is something that every woman looks forward too-- NOT!!! I was a little scared to have it done because my transplant incision is at the bottom of my breasts and goes from under one arm pit all the way across to the other arm pit. (They actually open you up like a clam). The only time it was painful is when they tried to get as close to the rib cage as possible. My rib cage is still sore from the car accident, my stupid fall, and a loose wire. But all in all, it wasn't as bad as I thought it was going to be.

This same morning when I was eating a bowl of raisin bran I cracked one of my teeth in half. I called my transplant coordinator, and she is sending me some penicillin pills that I am to take an hour before I go to the dentist. The pills won't be here until Friday when they are sending out the refill for the transplant drugs I'm on. I hope some of the pain goes away, because I won't be able to schedule an appointment until next week. They really don't want you to go to a dentist until you have reached a year since your Transplant. There can be so many bacterial infections in your mouth, that with a suppressed immune system you can easily pick up anything. But because the tooth is broken in half, if it is not taken care of, I could get a real bad infection. The tooth will have to be pulled, and then I suppose I'll have to wait until they can replace it with a crown.

So far, this has been a very busy week where you don't get a lot accomplished, but you do a lot of driving. I should say my husband did a lot of driving. The Doctor has now given me the o.k. to drive, but I'm still worried about getting behind the wheel again. (They say if you don't get back in the car, you never will). We have bought a car to replace the one I totaled. We bought a 2005 Ford Taurus SEL it only has 11,000 miles on it. It is in excellent shape, and I can't wait to be able just to get out of the house and go wherever I want. I have such an interesting life don't I? I really need help if all I'm looking forward to is getting out of the house!!

Chapter 49

My sister Linda used to work for Life Source, and they called her and asked her if I would give a speech to their employees about what my life was before the transplant, and what it is like now after the transplant. When Linda and I first discussed a transplant together, she explained Life Source to me. She explained that they were the people who work with the donor families. They totally support the family and collaborate with the transplant staff of the recipient, and set up the organ recovery process with the transplant team. They are the Link for the upper Midwest that matches the donor to the recipients. They are the Guardian Angels that turn "Loss into Life again."

My first response was, "What a horribly emotional job to have!" You would have to be a very compassionate person, and strong enough to handle so much grief. I have always considered myself a compassionate person, but I personally would not be strong enough to handle the grief. I'd be sitting with the family crying right along with them!! Their job is behind the scenes for the transplant recipient, but all of us who have had a transplant know that without their efforts and dedicated hard work they do with the families of the donors is what makes it all happen for us.

A lot of people used to believe (myself included) years ago, that if you were a donor, they wouldn't make much of an effort to keep you alive, because they wanted your organs!! (I think that line of thinking must have came from the movie (COMA).

Many more Transplants are being done today because of the great job that Life Source does to get the word out that organs are needed. When I talked to my own daughters about what they thought of being organ donors, they both showed me on their licenses that they already were organ donors. I am really proud of them for doing it on their own. So, when I renewed my license I signed up to be a donor. I only hope there is something good left of me to give.

When my sister Linda asked me to come and speak to them, I was very hesitant at first, because I don't usually speak in front of people I don't know very well, Even though I was a customer service manager and had to speak to many employees, that was different, because I knew them all, so I just thought pretend you know them all and you won't know when to shut-up! But I wouldn't have missed this opportunity to THANK THEM all personally for giving me back my life. Without the effort of the Univ. of Minn., Life Source, and my Donor (who will remain in my heart forever, even though we've never met) I will be eternally grateful to all of them.

THANK YOU ALL FROM THE BOTTOM OF MY HEART, OR IN MY CASE FROM THE BOTTOM OF MY LUNGS!!!

Our meeting with Life Source had to be re-scheduled. My sister Linda was going to do some painting, and she had recently bought a marble table which she thought she'd move out of the way and tip it over on it's top. Well the marble was not attached to the table, and when she went to tip it over it fell on her foot. She cut a few of her toes, smashed a toe, and ended up with three broken toes. As you know they cannot set a toe, so they wrapped her foot and she has to wear a boot.

Luckily, she lives really close to her work, so she is able to drive with her left foot, but she cannot take the chance of getting on the freeway. She has to wait six weeks before they can determine if she has to have surgery or not.

In the meantime we've-scheduled it for September 12. Let's hope we can make it this time. Of course if she has to have surgery on her foot, we will have to re-schedule it again. Hopefully it will heal properly on its own.

Chapter 50

We have a large oak tree that sits in our back yard down by the lake. It is starting to loose a lot of branches on it, so I wanted to call a tree service and have them come out and trimmed it, but I remember the last time I had a big oak tree trimmed. We also had a really large oak tree in our yard at our old home which was in desperate need of trimming. We hired a tree service that came out ant trimmed it up really nice. It really looked nice when they finished it.

The next day we had a tornado come through, and it up-rooted the tree and it fell on our home! Luckily, we had an older home that we had fully updated (almost 100 years old), so the framing on the house went from bottom to top and they were actually made with two by tens. Our insurance estimator that came out said we were very lucky that it was an older home otherwise with the newer homes, the tree would have went through the house and all the way to the basement. Instead it went through into the attic but didn't drop any farther. Because our home was a 4plex, it was two and a half stories high with a full attic. The only other thing on the house is that the tree branches went through the upstairs kitchen windows. Half of the tree root came out of the ground, and it was taller than I am. When the tree landed on our home, we felt the vibration and heard the noise, but didn't realize that the tree was down. Because this happened after dark, and of course when the storm hit, we had no power, we decided to deal with it in the morning. The next day we couldn't believe that the tree was on our home, and covered most of the house on that side. We also saw that the neighbor's smaller tree also up-rooted and it fell on our garage. The neighbors were extremely good about coming over and working to get their tree off of our garage. We called the insurance company right away, and they we're sending out an estimator as soon as they could that day. In the meantime my husband brewed a pot of coffee on the stove, and we decided to walk around the neighborhood to survey the damages. There was junk lying everywhere!! My husband's brother lived right next door to us, and he didn't suffer any damage at all. The rest of the neighborhood looked like a war zone. The neighbor had set up her Garage the day before for a sale. What was really funny, is that the garage had been lifted off its foundation, and landed smashed in the neighbor's yard, but all the stuff she had set on tables were not disturbed in any way!!

As we we're walking around, we must have been asked at least ten times where we had gotten the coffee from since we had no electricity? MY husband told them that we and they still had gas, so we brewed a pot on the stove with our camping peculator. (Most of them still didn't get it by the look on their faces)! On the way home, I happened to look at the top of our building, and I said to my husband "where is our chimney?"

He went up on the roof, and found it laying up there it had been broken off. The insurance company called a tree service to cut all the branches off the tree, and then they called a crane service to remove the tree off of our home. (We sure drew a crowd to witness that event)! I talked to the gentleman that was operating the crane, and I explained to him that since he was there could he also lift our chimney off of the roof, otherwise I didn't know how we were going to get it down. But he was very obliging and also removed the chimney at no extra charges. The only problem we had with our insurance is that since only one side of the house was damaged, they would only pay to replace that siding. Wouldn't you know it, they no longer made the exact color of steel siding that we had, so it was darker than the rest of the house.

Our youngest Granddaughter would be very happy to see this tree gone, because she does not like it. It has two large branches that are extended out and it looks like the tree has arms. When it is storming outside she won't even look out the window because she is afraid of it. I was thinking about going out and buying one of those sets of tree faces where the eyes light up, (but even I can't be that mean) so I figured I had better not or she'll never come to Grandmas house again!!

Chapter 51

This past year has been very good, and also very bad. Great things happened (Transplant) but also bad things have happened. (Accident). I received the results of my mammogram the other day and an abnormality was found in my right breast. They said it was non cancerous, so I just have to wait six months, then go in for an ultra sound. My transplant coordinator also called and said that the wrong lab instructions were sent with my lab mailers, so she has to send me out new ones, and I will have to have the tests repeated. I have been able to have these labs done at the hospital where I usually go to so at least I don't have to drive all the way to the U. But I have to call her back, and see if she can add a kidney function test to the labs, because my ankles are starting to swell, and I know its not my glucose, because that has been running low.

I cannot wait for this year to end!! I am looking forward to see what the New Year will bring. Since I've had my transplant I signed up to be in two study groups. One of these studies can't help me. but it can help people down the line with their transplants. The first one is when I have my bronscopy done they put in a little extra fluid then they take it back out and it goes to them. They are doing a study to see what they can find out and they're trying to make it possible for people not to have to go through so many bronscopy's in the first year. (That would be great for them, because right now you have to do at least six.) .The second study group is for doing a Spirometry at home every day. This test consists of breathing into a tube which monitors your air volume. This is to help them see any abnormalities (like rejection) before your monthly doctor visits. I have received a very nice letter from them telling me that they appreciate my hard work and dedication to this study. I have done it the most of anyone else in this study and they really appreciate my perseverance and commitment. But I don't see how the people who joined up for this wouldn't be doing it as much as they possibly can, because it's also very vital for them. I keep track of all the results myself. Of course I'm not a doctor so I have no idea if my lungs are doing really great, or if I need to put more effort into my therapy!! I suppose I could show my doctor the chart I made out the next time I see him, and he can let me know if my lungs are doing as well as they should be 5 ½ months after surgery.

Chapter 52

I went back to Dr. D. for my monthly check-up for my lungs. I had forgotten all about my second fall, but my daughter had driven me to the hospital, so she made sure that she told him about it. (that will be the last time SHE goes with me). But actually, I really did forget. My husband is in the process of changing the shutters on the house with the new color I wanted. I thought I would help him by taking off the kitchen shutters because they are on first floor. The window is not very high off the ground, so all I had to do was go up two rungs on the ladder. I had forgotten all about the fact that wasps like to build their nests behind the shutters, so when I started to take the first screw out a wasp flew out of the shutter right towards my face. Of course I backed up, but I forgot I was on a ladder, so I fell backwards and landed flat on my back. I laid on the ground for a little bit to see if I had any pain radiating from anyplace in my body, but everything seemed fine. He ordered another CT scan to see how the other pool of fluid looked and they discovered another new pool of fluid. Now they have two to keep an eye on. He said that if I didn't stay off of ladders he would take all my privileges away before I get a chance to kill myself. So I had better start doing as he says, and be more careful and quit doing things just because I can! I informed him that my mammogram came back showing a couple nodules, so I have to go back in six months to have an ultra sound done. He asked me if I had seen my doctor before I had the mammogram for an exam, and when I told him no, that I just set up the test because it was due, he said that he didn't want me to wait six months that I was to call and make a doctor appointment and have the ultra sound done sooner. So I made the appointment with her, she also felt the nodules, so she set me up for an ultra sound the next day. After the ultra sound was done, the radiologist came in and informed me that there were a couple nodules in the right breast and that he would let my doctor know so that they could set me up for a biopsy or to surgically have them removed. I didn't think Dr. D would go for the surgery part, because they wouldn't want to have me opened up. If they don't want you going to the Dentist, it would have to be very critical before they'd consent to surgery. They set me up for a consultation with a surgeon, and he and Dr. D decided on the biopsies.

The same radiologist that I had seen the first time did the biopsies. He asked me if I wanted a sedative before he began. I asked him if I would have to stay longer because of it, and do most women take a sedative? He said that yes I would have to stay in recovery a while, and that most women did choose the sedative, but I told him I drove myself, so I had better not. He told me to start talking to him about anything, so it took my mind off of what he was doing. He never should have asked me that because I start talking and never shut up. A couple of times he had to wait to continue because I had him laughing. He knows Dr. D because he used to work with him at the university. He said that I had better quit being so honest with him, and if there ever is another accident to make up a good story as to why the accident happened. He said that the next time, to tell him that I hit the tree because **I dropped my beer when I was trying to light a cigarette.** (I really laughed hard at that because after you've had a transplant you cannot ever have alcohol, or smoke)!!) He was a fantastic Dr. before I knew it, the biopsies were done and he sure did a great job of taking my mind off of the procedure. I told you that I couldn't wait for this year to end. I also had my bronscopy done and everything is continuing to look good. I only have three months more to wait and they can decrease my antibiotics from two to one. Then hopefully after a year, I can stop taking that antibiotic.

Chapter 53

Every time I go to the university I run into someone who had their transplant the same week I did. It's interesting to see how they are adjusting, and what problems they are having. This last time I ran into the young lady who had her Transplant done the same day as I did. She had her Transplant for Cystic Fibrosis, and she had a lot of set backs also. She ended up being in the hospital until June. You sure wouldn't know it by looking at her now. She looks fantastic, and she is starting College this week. I hope she continues to get better and better.

One of the other women who had her transplant the same week, I used to see her almost every time I was there, but I haven't seen her in a while. I knew she went home, someplace south of the cities. But I figured she had to come to the university also for her check-ups. When I received my new transplant letter I found out why I haven't seen her, she had died in June. I really felt bad she was always so up beat and positive about everything, and she leaves behind a teenage son. It is so hard to believe that she has died. It makes you realize that your body can reject the new lungs at any time. You really hope and pray that after your transplant that you are able to live for a few years. But, only God knows how much time that any of us has left.

Everyone keeps telling me that God still has a purpose for me, and that is why I have survived all my setbacks. I have always believed in God and that when you die you go to a better place. But I must be in a state of depression, because now I'm thinking that when you die, you just cease to exist anymore. It would be just like going to sleep but never waking up again. Then I think about what Dr. Red had said in an article that was written about her that God has given her the capability to do what she does, and for this she makes sure that her butt is sitting in a pew every Sunday! Maybe I should follow her lead, and get myself back to church again, to see what I'm missing in my life. I really don't think I've totally lost my faith in God, but somehow I've wandered out of his sight and I need to be put back on the right direction. I have no reason to be depressed because God has given me my life back again, but then my brain thinks it needs proof of his existence, and I know that God wants us just to believe. They say that God never gives you more that you can handle, but faith doesn't get you around your problems, it takes you through them. I found this poem in a book my sister had given me about angels, the author is unknown.

WHISPER OF ANGEL WINGS

Today I stumbled and once again was lifted by an unseen hand.

What comfort and joy that knowledge brings.

For I hear the whisper of angels wings

The guardian angel God sends to us all, to bear us up when we stumble and fall.

Trust him my friend and often you will hear, the whisper of angel wings hovering near.

Chapter 54

Today is my Birthday (September 11) Happy Birthday Too ME. Since today is a Monday, we will wait to celebrate it until the kids come up. My husband and I did go out to supper, but other than that we did nothing special. Tomorrow is the day that I go to Life Source with my sister, and give a talk to the employees about my life before and after my transplant. I really do not like speaking in front of a bunch of people I don't know, but the work they do is so great I really do want to thank them personally for giving my life back to me.

My sister Linda used to work at Life source so she gave a speech before me to let them know how their efforts affected her life also, and she never knew she would also know what it is like to be a family member of a person needing a transplant. She was very professional with her speech, and I was trying to make my speech not so depressing by putting some humor in it. It went very well they actually all looked very interested in what I had to say. I only broke down twice (which I knew I would) but I regained myself and went on. They want me to give my speech to hospitals in my area, but I told them I would have to get back to them, because I don't want to plan anything until I get my biopsy results back..

It went better than I thought it would, and I received many compliments. Maybe this is the plan that God has for me, and that is to make people aware of the need for organ donations.

After we finished there, we went and picked up my sister Colleen (her Birthday is the day before mine) and we went to the Casino to have lunch and to celebrate our Birthdays. We even had supper at the casino, and we didn't leave there until after midnight! I'm not used to being out this late, so needless to say, I was just exhausted the next day. I was a regular couch potato! But we had a lot of fun so it was worth it.

Chapter 55

I finally received the results of my breast biopsies, and they did not find any cancer. It took so long to get the results I was starting to get a little worried. I have to have an ultra sound done in another six months, just to make sure they haven't gotten any larger, or no new nodules have developed. I still think it has something to do with where they cut me for my transplant, but I guess it's better to be safe than sorry, so the test is probably a good idea.

I also still haven't had my October Bronscopy done. My blood just does not want to cooperate and coagulate itself. We found this out at my last doctor appointment, so he put me on vitamin k for the next four days, then took the test again but instead of going down, my INR was higher than it was the first time. So they cancelled my Bronc. Again and he put me on vitamin K for a week, and then re-schedule my bronc. I went back the day before, and my blood still wasn't correct so once again they cancelled the Bronchoscope. I had some type of special test done, but that came out o.k. but my INR is still high. So today, I had to see my regular doctor to get a flu shot, so my transplant coordinator set up another special test, they should get the results in a couple of days, then they will decide if they will send me to a blood specialist, or figure out what to do next! The blood disorder specialist took a bunch of blood but she said I did not have a blood disorder that she just thinks it's just from my anemia.

Chapter 56

If it's something weird, of course my body is going to get it. I went and had a root canal done one year, and I woke up with the left side of my face and my neck all swollen. I went right in to see the dentist the next morning, and he sent me to an oral surgeon right away. The oral surgeon opened up my neck on the left side and put in a drainage tube. It only made it worse, so he put me in the hospital to see if they could pump a lot of antibiotics through me, and see if they could get the infection to clear. I was in the hospital for a couple of days, when they went back in, and drained a lot of the infection. The swelling started to go down but it was taking a while.

It was Christmas Eve, and I already had been in the hospital for two weeks, so I begged him to let me go home and be with my kids. He wasn't too positive about it, but he let me go home. I was feeling better in a couple of days, so I went back to work. Everything was fine until I ran out of antibiotics. He said I didn't need them refilled, because I had been on them long enough!

Well, about a week after I had finished the antibiotics I woke up with my face and neck starting to swell up again. I went right in to see the oral surgeon, and he suggested that those two teeth come out so the infection would go away and stay away. So I let him remove those two teeth. But it didn't help. The swelling was getting worse again. I was practically in tears when I went back to see him, and once again I was put back in the hospital. The infectious disease doctor suggested I have an MRI done so they could actually see what was going on.

Of course I had never had an MRI done, so when they wheeled me down to x-ray and I see this tube like machine with a door on it, I started to really panic! I told the doctor that I was very claustrophobic and there was NO WAY they were putting me in that tube, and shut the door on me. They explained the whole procedure to me but it didn't do anything to set my mind at ease. My doctor was called in, and he told me just to shut my eyes before I go in, and don't open them until I came out. So I said I would give it a try, but if I wanted OUT they had better let me out. Well I did exactly as he told me to do, and there was a fan blowing in there (Which helped) but I just kept trying to think of other things instead of what was going on.

But I think my blood pressure must have doubled because of my fears. I have never had another one, AND I NEVER WILL! They say now they have glass on both sides, but I don't care if there is glass on all four sides. You are still stuck in this tube with no way out! Funny, I'll go through a transplant, but I won't get an MRI. We all have certain fears, and some stay with us for a long time.

Chapter 57

I just finished writing a letter to the family of my donor. That was a very, very hard letter to write. I don't know why, but I think my donor was a he. I kept writing he then I had to go back and change it. It is so hard to say Thank You to the family of your donor because in order for you to still be here someone else had to die. But everyone keeps telling me that this person would have died whether they donated an organ or not, but that doesn't make it any easier on you.

You feel so much love and gratitude towards this person, and you know you will never be able to thank them personally. One part of you would really like to know everything about this person, but another part of you doesn't want to know the person who died to give you life. You have a lot of mixed feelings going on at this time your heart is suffering the loss of this person, but also the love you feel for this person.

Your brain wants to absorb all the information you can get on them. I really haven't decided if I want them to write back to me or not. I guess I should have waited to write my letter until I was sure, but I felt it was time I acknowledged this person to their family. I'm sure when the family gets my letter they will also have trouble deciding if they want to write back to me or not. But whatever they decide is alright because I will understand their feelings. It is a very hard choice to decide to write or not, but it has to be their choice. It is not easy to pour your heart out to someone you don't know.

This is a passage that I found while reading a book by Richard Eyre:

"Most of us know in our more introspective moments, that our deepest truest selves are noble and good. We are natural, physical people with countless faults, weaknesses, lusts, and appetites, and we are prone towards all kinds of mistakes. Yet, deep down our core is good."

In conclusion, let me say that all the pain and setbacks I suffered were worth it just too still be able to be here with my family. I really enjoyed writing this book I call my Journal, and I hope you enjoy reading it as much. I wanted to give everyone a better understanding of what it is like to be the recipient of a transplant. The whole experience was over whelming, and I hope you understand the benefit of putting "Donor" on your license. Everyone deserves a second chance at life, and we all need to get the word out that donor's are needed to give as many people as possible a second chance at life.

Who knows, it's only been nine months since my transplant, and I have a lot more memories stored in my brain, so maybe you will hear from me again.........God willing.

www.ingramcontent.com/pod-product-compliance
Ingram Content Group UK Ltd.
Pitfield, Milton Keynes, MK11 3LW, UK
UKHW020141250726
13967UKWH00002B/795

9 781425 172596